Why Can't We Sleep?

DARIAN LEADER

HAMISH HAMILTON
an imprint of
PENGUIN BOOKS

HAMISH HAMILTON

UK | USA | Canada | Ireland | Australia
India | New Zealand | South Africa

Hamish Hamilton is part of the Penguin Random House group of companies
whose addresses can be found at global.penguinrandomhouse.com.

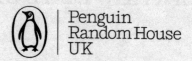

Penguin
Random House
UK

First published 2019
001

Copyright © Darian Leader, 2019

The moral right of the author has been asserted

Set in 11/13 pt Dante MT Std
Typeset by Jouve (UK), Milton Keynes
Printed and bound in Great Britain by Clays Ltd, Elcograf S.p.A.

A CIP catalogue record for this book is available from the British Library

ISBN: 978–0–241–98443–7

www.greenpenguin.co.uk

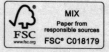

PENGUIN BOOKS

Why Can't We Sleep?

Darian Leader is a British psychoanalyst and the author of *Introducing Lacan*, *Why Do Women Write More Letters Than They Post?*, *Promises Lovers Make When It Gets Late*, *Freud's Footnotes*, *Stealing the Mona Lisa*, *Why do People Get Ill* (co-written with David Corfield), *The New Black*, *What Is Madness*, *Strictly Bipolar* and *Hands*. He practises psychoanalysis in London, and he is a member of the College of Psychoanalysts and a founding member of the Centre for Freudian Analysis and Research.

For Imre and Janet

Selling Sleep

'I am an excellent sleeper,' says Freud in *The Interpretation of Dreams*. Not everyone is so lucky. At least one in three adults complains of lack of sleep, and the prescription of sleeping pills has been increasing dramatically over the past few decades. Sleep clinics, which were once a rarity, are now a feature of most major hospitals, and in the United States can even be found in shopping malls and spas. People take pills not only to sleep but then to stay awake the next day, just as so many of us rely on coffee and energy drinks to maintain an artificial state of arousal during our waking hours. Once considered a natural state, sleep has now become a commodity, something that we must fight to acquire and which we are never quite sure of possessing.

Almost every day, newspapers, internet sites and TV shows spotlight some new story about sleep: how much of it we need, what will happen if we don't get it, how much the economy loses through tired workers. Sleep experts broadcast their advice and opinions, as if some new philosopher's stone has been found. Basic aspects of the human condition such as anxiety, sadness and failure are now presented as the consequences of a lack of nourishing sleep. Rather than seeing insomnia, for example, as the result of a depressive state, causality is inverted: we are depressed because we haven't slept.

Facts about sleep that have been known for more than

a hundred years are now being marketed as cutting-edge research. The link between sleep and memory was studied carefully in the nineteenth century, yet the old theories are back as if they have only just been discovered. This new excitement around sleep science will no doubt fade with time, yet we need to ask why it is happening now. Are we just so desperate to find some kind of universal explanation for our woes that we turn to the one part of human life that can't answer back? Or is there a new epidemic of sleep problems caused by the digital age we inhabit?

As we lie in bed, emails, texts and social media posts stack up, and it seems as if the demands of the outside world are limitless. Many people check their phones before going to sleep – and even during their sleep – and then reach for them again at the moment of waking. Sleep science tells us that the blue light from our screens will interfere with the process of falling asleep, but it is surely the demands themselves that have a greater effect. There is no let-up. We are continually being told things, shown things, asked things, obliged to do things – and reminded when we have failed to. Like the 'sleep mode' on our phones – which is a form of being 'on' – we are now never really able to be 'off'.

Does this mean that there is a new urgency to do precisely that: turn ourselves off? The irony here is that if we suffer from the fact that we can't stop the relentless chain of demands, sleeping has now been added to the list. It is as if a light bulb with an electrical current running through it is told to turn itself 'off' by the current itself. The constant flow of messages and imperatives that shape our environment is now bloated by the message to turn off the flow. Where spas and wellness centres were once the destination where privileged people were supposed to go to find peace, it is now sleep itself that is marketed as one's own individual retreat.

The economic opportunities here are substantial. If spas were for the wealthy few, sleep is for everyone, rich and poor alike. Adverts for mattresses, once a rarity, now regularly punctuate commercial breaks and web feeds, and the sleep aid industry will generate an estimated $76.7 billion this year alone. If one early study at Edinburgh University in the 1950s claimed that there wasn't that much difference in sleep time between using a wooden board and a fancy sprung mattress, today the dull rectangle is sold as the necessary gateway into sleep. Your insomnia is caused less by your worries than by the fact that your mattress is not gold standard.

This burgeoning of the mattress industry is made possible by the powerful pressure put on us to sleep in the right way. Just as the media constantly tell us what food we should eat and what exercise we should take, we are now instructed on how and when we must sleep. And the more that such norms are disseminated, the more that deviations from them become seen as 'disorders' or 'illnesses'. If a few decades ago there were only a handful of sleep disorders that one could suffer from, today there are more than seventy. And with more disorders come more cures, more experts, more revenue.

What gets forgotten here is both obvious and invisible. We can be told how we must sleep, but not how to process the instruction itself. If we read an article that explains why an eight-hour sleep is essential for our health and advises us on what to do to achieve this, won't the pressure to sleep correctly actually get in the way of our sleep? This is indeed what insomniacs have been telling us for many years: the more we are enjoined to focus on sleep, the thought itself will keep us awake. And yet we live in a world where we are relentlessly coerced to live healthily, to manage our bodies, to do our best to sleep deeply and restoratively.

On waking, it is this imperative that greets us, as we calculate how long we have succeeded in sleeping. For those who believe in human evolution, the image is sobering: where perhaps centuries ago we might have woken from sleep and begun the tasks of the day, now we wake up and check a clock, to measure our sleeping hours against a norm. And the more there is a norm, the more there will be those who fail to fit it. The diversity that we are supposed to celebrate elsewhere is expunged here, as variations in how we sleep become disorders of sleep. Many people thus wake to a sense of failure, starting their day with an internal judgement that they have not succeeded in a task, and worrying about how this will affect them.

The calculus of self-reproach and salvation that the new health discourse creates echoes uncannily the role that the Church once played. Just as the Church's prescriptions would directly impact ways of life, shaping both the psyche and the flesh with its codes of conduct and judgement, so today we change the ways we live and think according to what we learn from biomedicine, the dominant belief system of the Western world. How much fruit we eat, how we exercise and how we sleep are to a large extent influenced by this discourse. And where the Church would count sins and transgressions, so we count our pieces of fruit, our laps, our steps and our hours of sleep.

Just as theologians would debate endlessly the validity of their spiritual quantifications, so today the thresholds for vitamin intake, pieces of fruit, hours of sleep, cholesterol and blood pressure have been frequently redefined. Whatever the validity of such shifts, don't they testify to a basic wish to define the body using numbers? Don't we want a hard and fast number to serve as a dividing line between health and illness, between right and wrong? There is an assumption here that applying numbers to the body confers some kind of truth to the claims, even if we then find that they are almost always questioned or revised.

After several years of being told to eat five pieces of fruit and vegetables, new research claimed that the figure should in fact be ten. But there is quite a big difference between five and ten. Revisions of such magnitude rarely dent people's faith in modern science, although the history of both science and medicine is filled with quite radical recalculations, from the age of the universe, to the amount of dark matter, to the ratio of neuroglial cells to neurons, all of which have been increased by more than a factor of two. Yet imagine if the sleep scientists were to tell us that eight was wrong, and that we actually needed sixteen hours of sleep each night.

Eight is certainly a magic number. It divides nicely into twenty-four, and has been linked to sleep for centuries, advocated by both Maimonides and Alfred the Great. The latter's famous candle clock partitioned the day into a third for reading, writing and prayer, a third for conducting the business of the realm and a third for 'the refreshment of the body'. Yet, as one sixteenth-century physician could write, 'Old ancient doctors of physic say 8 hours of sleep in summer and 9 in winter is sufficient for any man, but I do think that sleep ought to be taken as the complexion of man is.' Individual variation has always been recognised, yet it is only in more recent times that our worries are both shaped and accentuated by the numerical norm.

Not only are we instructed to sleep for eight hours, but the magic number is now being used to sell the very beds that we sleep in. As the writer Jon Mooallem puts it, whereas mattresses were once 'anonymous white rectangles', today they have become 'holistic health and wellness machines'. No one really bothered to regularly change these cumbersome slabs, yet we are now pressured to do so . . . every eight years! The association of this number with a marketing campaign draws on the very conditioning that is arguably a part of falling asleep. Just as preparing for bed because we are tired may mean becoming tired because we are preparing for bed, so the number that represents a good night's sleep becomes the sign of the right moment to buy a new mattress.

This form of conditioning is both carefully exploited and magically ignored in much of today's sleep science. Books and scholarly articles explain, for example, the obstructive effect of alcohol, and state that the habit of the bedtime tipple will compromise rather than ensure a good night's sleep. Yet what of the drinker's association of the drink with sleep? The effect of this conditioning – which can be robust – is entirely forgotten, yet the very same sleep science can then advocate cognitive therapies for insomnia that rely precisely on a conditioning process. These therapies are helpful to many people, and involve associating certain patterns of behaviour with going to sleep.

Curiously, where hygiene books of the 1950s were declaring that everyone needed eight hours of sleep, popular science tomes of the 1960s saw this as what the sleep researcher William Dement termed a 'fallacy', and it was widely ridiculed. As two American writers on sleep pointed out in 1968: 'With so many factors co-determining onset, amount and depth of sleep in various individuals, the physician cannot indiscriminately demand of each patient that he go to bed early, fall asleep promptly, or generally, sleep quantitatively "by the book", and then translate such expectations into a routinized medicinal regimen. In fact, one may say that overconcern with the problem of sleep and its individual variations is a symptom which sometimes afflicts both patient and physician and is, in some ways, as serious as the condition with which it concerns itself.' The writers are incredulous that anyone can still believe in an 'eight-hour law' where each of us can spend our nights in a 'delightful oblivion', yet this is precisely what many of today's sleep hygienists tell us we need.

Drug companies take out ads to alert people that they may have a sleep disorder and require medication if they don't get their sleep hours, lacking the energy to do the things they need to do, such as spend time with their family or perform their duties at work, or if they experience mental tiredness, body fatigue, low motivation and difficulty concentrating. Yet as sleep historian Matthew Wolf-Meyer observes, aren't these symptoms the very conditions of modern life, and indeed, of life as it has been lived for centuries? And when an advert for a mattress company begins by asking viewers if they find themselves unable to concentrate during the day, have problems remembering things and use a lot of clichés when they speak, rather than seeing this as a consequence of the pressures of modern life, long commutes and an unbearable exhortation to maintain a positive image during working hours, it is declared the sign of a poor mattress.

The description given of the sleep-deprived individual in fact pretty much suits most people today in urban society. Yet rather than recognising the effects of socio-economic burdens and internal pain, human difficulties are redefined through the new lens of unbroken sleep. When we forget or fail, it is because we did not wake up feeling happy and refreshed after a great sleep. In one of the most celebrated stories of forgetfulness, King Alfred was on the run from the Vikings and took shelter in the home of a poor peasant. After she asked him to keep an eye on the cakes while she attended to some chores, his mind wandered and on her return she found them burnt to a crisp. How long will it be before a sleep hygienist claims that the distracted king's inattentiveness was actually the result of sleep deprivation, due to a failure to get the eight hours he had himself recommended? If he had slept right, he would have performed better, and left England without the legacy of burnt cakes that it is still trying to correct with its *Bake Offs*.

Losing Sleep

Sleep science began in the late nineteenth century, was fractured by the First World War, and then expanded during the twentieth century, accelerating from the 1960s onwards. Electroencephalography – the measurement of electrical potentials in the brain – allowed different stages of neural activity to be distinguished during sleep, although no theory was able to explain adequately what they represented. The widely publicised link between the rapid eye movement stage of sleep (REM) and dreaming in the early 1950s led to a mass of new research and funding, yet by the early 80s, dreaming was no longer central to the agenda. The emphasis would move away from the psychological phenomena to what appeared to be the purely physical, focusing on research into body clocks, the neural and neurochemical basis of sleep and its disorders, and the study and treatment of apnoea, the temporary suspension of breathing during sleep.

Although today's sleep science is obviously a complex field, with many different research areas, two features stand out when we compare it with the earliest work. First of all, sleep has moved away from the individual's experience to become an objectified, external object. Sleep journals today won't quote the words of patients, and experiences with labels like 'insomnia' are very rarely dependent on how the person actually describes them. The historian Kenton Kroker calls his study of sleep science *The Sleep of Others* to stress how sleep was progressively taken away from the individual and transformed into a new artefact that could be manipulated and dissected with no reference to introspection.

Secondly, from the late 1920s on, sleep research would become much more of a player in the economic marketplace than it had been previously. Research was – and continues to be – substantially funded by business and the military, with the aim of maximising the efficiency and productivity of workers and soldiers. Even the idea of a single unit of sleep is a relatively recent invention, the historians tell us, dating back probably only a couple of hundred years. Prescriptive notions of sleep became widespread during and after the Industrial Revolution, with the implementation of the factory day in the 1840s.

Workers were expected to labour for between twelve and sixteen hours, settling into the eight-hour working day in the twentieth century in many Western cultures. The eight-hour day is, of course, a relative luxury, and most of the world's population still work for much longer than this. The figures for work and rest were set not by a concern with anyone's well-being but by the demands of factory schedules and production processes that the new technologies introduced. Continuous and unbroken performance became the ideal that workers had to aspire to.

The growth of industries such as oil and steel, which require twenty-four-hour production, needed workers who had enough sleep to function effectively. Sleep, with the expansion of industry, was quantified as an adjunct to work, and the minimum time necessary had to be carefully calculated. Nathaniel Kleitman, widely considered to be one of the founders of sleep science in the twentieth century, would publish his vast academic study *Sleep and Wakefulness* in 1939, and then follow it up with a summary in the popular magazine *American Business*. His University of Chicago research was heavily funded by corporate sponsors keen to engineer more productive workers, and he would even feed pureed beef to five-week-old babies after the local meat business Swift and Co. gave $10,000 to try to show that they would sleep better on a bovine-filled stomach.

Sleep here is something to be manipulated and crafted, with the aim not of improving people's lives but of increasing productivity, or, in the case of the military, training soldiers who can stay awake for days with the minimum sleep possible. During the Vietnam War, massive quantities of amphetamines were dispensed by the US Army to keep its troops awake, and more recently, it began the Continuous Assisted Performance project, aiming to eliminate the need for sleep temporarily through drugs and electrical stimulators. Many sleep scientists today are quite happy to take the cheque from such sponsors, giving workshops for bank executives on the optimal ways to rest and access the sleep that less privileged employees and outsourced labour are unlikely ever to enjoy.

Even the most disinterested and well-intentioned sleep research posits as a benchmark 'optimal performance', as if human beings are ultimately workers who must be made – or allowed – to function as fruitfully as possible. If you don't get your eight hours, you will underperform, failing at physical and cognitive tasks that a good night's sleep should have made effortless.

The idea that underperformance could itself actually be a benchmark seems unthinkable.

———

As for the extraction of sleep from the individual's own experience, this is something that insomniacs are familiar with. Wired up to track brain wave patterns, breathing, heart rate, eye movement and muscle activity, technicians can show that the three-hour sleep complained of was in fact five or six hours. Tracking devices used at home can produce similar discrepancies, indicating that the time spent awake was far less than the person imagined. But aren't we dealing here with two entirely different times?

What the apparatus fails to factor in is a difference between clock time and subjective time. A measuring device cannot record how long a person experiences wakefulness. When sleep scientists tell us with a smile that insomniacs nearly always overestimate the time they lie awake, this is a mistake, because the two metrics at play here are incommensurable. The person may be persuaded that when they thought they were awake they were in fact asleep, drawn into error by the high frequency of microarousals during certain phases of sleep, but this is to gloss over the problem. The sleep scientist does not have an instrument to measure subjective time, since this is, by definition, the time that we experience, in which minutes can be felt like hours, and hours like endless days. Scientific-sounding labels like 'sleep state misperception' are only symptomatic of this impotence. What the insomniac and the sleep scientist mean by the word 'sleep' is not the same thing.

A patient described his many visits to doctors and sleep specialists, whom he had consulted over a period of several years. When he was finally able to spend a night in a sleep lab, he learnt that he was in fact sleeping for around six hours, and that his despair at what seemed to be an interminable night awake was unfounded. But being told this was unhelpful. Rather than bringing relief, it just compounded his anxiety. As he described his feelings, it became clear that what mattered for him was not only being able to sleep but a *recognition* that he was not sleeping. He had been brought up by a single mother, and when she started a relationship with a man when he was ten, he would lie awake, desperate not to hear any sound of them having sex. Silence was more terrifying than any external noise here, as he anticipated that it could be broken at any moment.

As he lay in bed, he would try to distance and suppress the hostile thoughts that came into his mind. He would reproach himself too for being capable of harbouring negative feelings towards someone he was supposed to love. When he eventually left home to pursue his studies, his sleep became easier, and the insomnia was only to emerge, years later, when a new partner moved in with him, bringing with her a son from a previous relationship. Now the triangle of his late childhood was re-established: a man and a woman sleep together, while a child lies in bed in an adjacent room.

The painful dilation of time that he experienced was not clock time, not a time that could be measured in minutes and hours, but the time of waiting for a sound that would petrify him. This was a time in which he was alone with his thoughts, oscillating between rage and self-blame. No one seemed to care about what he felt, and there was no one to acknowledge the dreadful new situation he was in when his mother began her relationship. Indeed, everyone around them was delighted, and he felt obliged to rejoice with them the changed circumstances. In his consultations all those years later, he sought, at some level, an authentification of his feelings, of what it had been like to lie there in that endless nocturnal limbo.

—

Those disciplines that do privilege listening over measuring have never come up with an overarching explanation of sleeping problems. In the talking therapies, it is rare for insomnia to be presented as the initial reason for consultation, though sleep difficulties will often then become apparent later on. In the case described above, I had no idea about them until quite a few months into our work. Given the agonies of insomnia, it is a question why this should be so. Is it that we simply need the right pointers to be able to speak about it, or, on the contrary, could there be a function in this avoidance?

With children, sleep difficulties are more transparent, probably because in most cases it is the parents who are woken up when their child cannot sleep, and it is they and not the child who then seek help. We often find that the child's sleep cannot be initiated due to a preoccupation with mortality or the body. 'How can I sleep,' they say, 'if I might never wake up?' after learning not long before that death is like a 'long sleep'. Even in the early twentieth century, a common bedtime prayer for children featured the clause 'If I should die before I wake'. Or, when nappies are on the way out, a fear of soiling the bedclothes may obstruct the sleep process. Bed-wetting, which was once seen as 'the most prevalent childhood sleep disorder', may thus give rise to its own, secondary 'disorder'.

The fairy tale of the princess and the pea gives a good model of this kind of precise and transitory disturbance of sleep. The poor protagonist is unable to fall asleep properly due to the pea placed beneath her mattresses, proof that she is in fact a real princess. Yet beneath the story is no doubt the narrative of sexual awakening: the little pea-shaped object keeps her awake at night, and sleep will come when the excitement at feeling it – or the guilt that this generates – is somehow processed. The story ends, indeed, with marriage to a prince, and hence the idea that a husband might take the place of the pea.

Traumatic experiences of all sorts can not only block sleep for a child but also wake them up in panic. A four-year-old girl would sit bolt upright in bed screaming, tearing at her arms even when her mother rushed to her and held her. In these night terrors, not uncommon in early childhood, the crisis continues beyond the moment of waking, and no comfort from the caregiver registers for several minutes, as if they are still within their trauma even when their eyes are wide open. In this instance, the source of the sleep disturbance seemed clear: the girl had been hospitalised two years previously in an emergency, and nurses had attempted to forcibly insert a cannula into both of her arms as she screamed in fear and agony. Later, in the night terror, she was there again, trying to tear the cannulas out of her arms.

Such cases of punctual and precise interruptions of

sleep are, in later life, more the exception than the rule. With children they tend to resolve swiftly, with or without therapeutic intervention, although they may prove more refractory when the anxieties of the parent become compounded with those of the child. It is very common, for example, for a parent to check on their sleeping child to make sure that they are not dead, even once the child is well beyond their first year. Similarly, bedclothes may be scrutinised minutely for any sign of effluvia or bodily deposit, as if the parent's own panic at staining and dirt cannot be separated off.

Yet we find again and again that the child's sleep symptoms settle over time, as they create other ways of elaborating the questions that preoccupy them. Playing, reading, drawing, daydreaming and talking all offer potential ways to symbolise and inscribe the fears and anxieties that surround sleep. The emergence of bedtime rituals in the second and third year is perhaps the most obvious treatment of these issues, as if the child places repetitive and sequential behaviours at the maximal point of psychological and physiological weakness, the transition between waking and sleep.

With adults, insomnia tends to be more complex. Although there are cases where its sudden appearance is clearly linked to a single cause which can then be unpacked, most of the time, when it is a chronic difficulty, several factors are at play. Many different problems are absorbed in what seems to be one monolithic symptom. Direct approaches are often fruitless here, and when the insomnia fades away, clinicians report that it is the result not of some immediate illumination or insight but rather, on the contrary, of a retroactive perception.

The patient will say one day that, strangely enough, they are now sleeping much better.

In the case we discussed earlier, linking the start of the insomnia with the new domestic triangle was crucial, and it opened up an exploration of the patient's past, but it did not produce any miraculous change in his sleeping difficulties. This would come much later, as he grappled with the question of his relation with his biological father. He had only met him a handful of times, and had always sided with his mother and her condemnation of an apparently brutal and uncaring man. When he learnt that his father was dying of a terminal illness, he had the opportunity to visit him but chose not to, yet after the death he began to doubt his decision. Had his mother been right? Did he not owe a duty to this man who had, after all, been 'one half of the reason why I exist'?

The dreadful night-time space of his insomnia would become like a punishment for him, as if he had to pay a price for his neglect. What the case shows so clearly is how several factors are at play in the sleeping problem: the insomnia was created, in a sense, by the childhood situation of staying awake at night listening apprehensively for sounds of his mother and her partner, and yet it would then come to take on a further function. As a receptacle for his self-accusations and the damages that they entailed, it had become the matrix of different forms of pain, doubt and sadness.

A sensitivity to these individual, specific causes of insomnia is becoming more and more difficult today in a society that privileges normative views of sleep. Just as we are told how much we need to sleep, so we are also often told what is stopping us from sleeping, from the blue light of our computers, to our poor scheduling of sleep, to the caffeine that we ingest. Some of this information is no doubt helpful – as are some of the recommended therapies – but we lose out on the narrative of individual lives and how this can clarify the sources of each person's difficulty with sleep.

In the last decade or so a new gloss has been added to this. Although the basic focus for sleep research remains that of productivity and efficacity, more and more attention is being paid to the effects of sleep loss on the health of the body. Cancer, heart disease, diabetes and endocrine problems are all being linked to inadequate sleep, with lack of sleep now identified as the 'silent killer' that heart disease once was. Some of these claims are persuasive and the research convincing, but what is interesting here is the way in which health can be superimposed so easily on the older imperatives to be productive.

Staying alive is today seen as a personal choice, a duty we must continually work at, so that existing is now just as much a task or product of our efficiency as work used to be. 'You must be as productive as possible' and 'You must stay alive as long as possible' increasingly mean one and the same thing. And with this the difference between health and illness becomes closer and closer to that between right and wrong, so that avoiding illness and remaining alive take on a moral value.

When a sleep hygienist declares that sleep will keep you slim, lower food cravings, protect you from cancer and dementia, lower the risk of heart disease, stroke and diabetes, and make you happier, more honest – yes, seriously – and less anxious, they add that the great thing about this is that it's all free. But the problem is that it is only – potentially – free if you do not happen to be like more than 95 per cent of the world's population, who have to struggle to make a living, keep long working hours, worry about their loved ones and the demands of employers, and achieve access to basic amenities. Many sleep hygienists dispense advice that is only for a privileged elite, where each individual has their own bedroom with sensitive temperature control and software that will tailor the environment to their unique circadian rhythm, waking them to artificial bursts of blue light that will make them happier and more hopeful in the morning.

But will pressure on poor people to sleep like the rich make their sleep any better? It might seem good news that US insurance giant Aetna, which has almost 50,000 employees, gives them a bonus for getting more sleep, based on a sleep tracker they can wear, yet this neglects to factor in the human costs of what it means to not get a bonus, and the pressures that reward systems introduce. If workers receive a $25-per-night bonus if they manage to sleep twenty seven-hour nights or more, what is really being introduced here if not the pressure to sleep more, to earn more, to earn as much as one's colleagues, and to be monitored even at night-time by one's employer? If you have trouble sleeping, don't worry, as once your sleep tracker identifies you as insomniac, you could receive cognitive therapy via your smartphone which will help you sleep healthily.

In this market-driven vision of the future, some sleep

scientists advocate sleep breathalysers in cars, which would prevent you embarking on your journey if a scanner identified you as having not had the required sleep. If it is true that one in two adults fails to get the sleep that they should, this might do wonders for global pollution, but of course it fails to factor in the effects of the rage and frustration that someone would feel if their car refused to start. Although so many traffic accidents are indeed caused by fatigue, it would be unwise to ignore the violence that car deprivation may involve, especially when we consider what a car might mean to its owner.

We could also pause here to reflect on the epidemiological data that links the hour shift when the clocks go forward in spring to a significant increase in car accidents the following Monday morning. Are these, after all, direct effects of fatigue and hence poor control of the vehicle due to the loss of an hour of sleep, or, on the contrary, due to increased anger, irritability and frustration as the person wakes up at the wrong time or feels robbed of precious sleep time? The human experience of clock change must surely be included in the equation here.

One Sleep or Two?

The emphasis on performance and productivity that now regulates sleep is often taken to have superseded the cycles of day and night that supposedly organised society prior to the Industrial Revolution. This is also the moment when two forms of time were separated from each other. As the social historian E. P. Thompson argued, it was during the Industrial Revolution that time became something to be *spent* rather than something to be passed: it became currency. Whereas in the pre-industrial era, the work pattern moved between intense labour and idleness focused around specific tasks, Thompson thought that it was now reoriented away from finite tasks to time itself, which could not be wasted.

Human beings no longer shared one and the same time, as there was now a difference between the time of the worker and the time of the master. Workers' time at rest was a master's time lost. When the worker was absent from the factory, this was the master's time spent, a division that would be internalised by the worker him- or herself. Uniform working hours and the monetarisation of time would be accentuated by the spread of timekeeping devices as well as public clocks. The time of industry, of nascent though not perfected capitalism, meant that the clocks changed: this was less the loss of an hour in summertime – adopted by many countries in the late nineteenth and early twentieth centuries – than the loss of a whole way of experiencing time itself.

When today's insomniac is told that they overestimate their time awake, are we not dealing with a form of this very division of time? There are two times here, one of which is dominant and 'correct', and the other relegated to the vagaries of individual perception. This is, after all, a clash of two discourses, two ways of seeing and of being in the world. However we want to gloss it, as the uneducated and misguided patient or as the mature and rational sleep expert, it is the difference between the time of the slave and the time of the master. To function correctly in society, we need to stick to the master's time.

The split between two times has indeed often been a symbol of social and political divisions. In his *Arcades Project*, Walter Benjamin cites a poetic depiction of the July revolution in Paris: 'Who would believe it! It is said that, incensed at the hour, / Latter-day Joshuas, at the foot of every clocktower, / Were firing on clock faces to make the day stand still.' The authors append a note to claim that this was a unique feature of the insurrection, 'the only act of vandalism carried out by the people against public monuments. And what vandalism! How well it expresses the situation of hearts and minds on the evening of the twenty-eighth!' This action was observed, we read, 'at the very same hour, in different parts of the city', and hence could not be taken for 'an isolated whim, but a widespread, nearly general sentiment'.

This division of times also marks some of the sleep science that documents circadian rhythms, the cycles regulated by internal body clocks that move along a roughly twenty-four-hour cycle. External cues known as zeitgebers – such as light, temperature and social interaction – help set or 'entrain' the circadian cycle, which is why night-shift work and flying across different time zones can have such deleterious effects on our sleep. Looking at graphs of circadian peaks and slumps during the course of the day and night, we find that human life is often divided between 'working' and 'sleeping', as if no other time is either present or possible.

The French use the expression 'Métro, boulot, dodo' – 'Tube, work, sleep' – to indicate a lifeless, automated existence, yet this is what the graphs of circadian rhythm presuppose, with no registration of napping habits, for example, or variation in sleep patterns. The division of the day into work and sleep is of course exactly what factory owners introduced, and one wonders how such results would appear when mapped onto the more complex realities of a human day. It is commonplace, after all, to try to create more time, especially through the use of chemical transitions: a drink to mark the end of a work day, or in the liminal time that so many of us introduce to border sleep, often staying up later and later just in order to do this.

A patient explained how she would create this private margin not late at night but in the small hours of the morning. Waking deliberately at 3 a.m., she would write her journal, snack and read, before returning to bed and then waking conventionally at 7.30 with her flatmates, who were totally unaware of her practice. She derived a satisfaction from their ignorance, as if she had created a double life, 'a time that belongs to no one else', as she put it. The more that we live to the time of others, with their schedules and urgencies, the more that this appeal to a solitary time becomes important, and once it is established, it can come to house a variety of activities that now take on a special value.

These times may be at odds with the circadian rhythms that contribute to our sleep–wake cycles, in the same way that they are contrary to the sleep requirements of late capitalism. The discovery of circadian rhythms was in itself coherent with the modern marketplace, since it showed that the body possessed sequencing that was not entirely dependent on the rising and setting of the sun. This meant that such rhythms could be explored in the context of an optimisation of a worker's productivity, and implied a disconnection between the individual and the social body, echoed in the distinction between the rhythm itself – purely endogenous – and the environmental cues – the zeitgebers – that helped set it.

Historians claim that circadian rhythms were to shift slightly in the nineteenth century, in part as an effect of the omnipresence of artificial lighting. The body was thus open to external intervention, and we can note how the language we use to speak of our relation to technology would come to apply to ourselves: like a clock or a meter, our biology can be 'reset'. Curiously, the wake–sleep cycle seems the most well-known physiological rhythm here, though several hundred bodily functions exist that oscillate between maximal and minimal values during the course of a day, and recent research has shown that almost every cell of the body operates with some form of timekeeping.

Logically, indeed, the incursion of the marketplace into sleep time had to happen. It made no sense that what was supposed to take up a third of human life could go unmonetarised, and the ancient practice of selling sleep potions and remedies would become the big business of the late nineteenth and twentieth centuries. Tech, pharma and mattress firms have invested heavily in advertising campaigns for their products. New algorithms and sleep-tracking devices promise to quantify sleep and its quality, and we are encouraged to be as worried about our night-time performance as our daytime activities. When sleep was linked with memory consolidation – which we will explore later on – time spent sleeping could be exploited in just this way, and sleep-teaching devices, which repeated words and information that the worker could master in his or her slumber, were once widely marketed.

The question of tracking – and surveillance – is usually taken to be benign here, allowing us to manage and improve ourselves. Some of the new mattresses come with built-in technology that will accrue data on its owner's sleep, and in many cases also follows the market's equation of size with value. Just as a Big Mac is better than a simple burger, so the new mattresses come with double, triple and quadruple layers of foam and fabric. Where in the fairy tale the multiplication of mattresses is a bizarre and obtrusive part of a test of royal lineage, today it becomes the supersized requirement for a good night's sleep.

If the time allotted to sleep was to become more and more fixed from the early nineteenth century, so was the very form of sleep itself. In an influential series of articles, and a book, *At Day's Close*, the historian Roger Ekirch has argued that the basic form of human sleep prior to this period was biphasic. Rather than one single consolidated block, humans had a first and then a second sleep. Retiring around 9 or 10 p.m., they would sleep till midnight or 1 a.m., then rise for an hour or two – in a period known as 'watching', which meant less 'looking' than 'being awake' – before returning to their 'second sleep' till morning. Although the times for starting the first and second sleeps would shift historically and geographically, the biphasic pattern was more or less constant.

Different cultures and times would have different ways of understanding this division of sleep, just as the activities to fill the gap between the two sleeps would vary. These might involve sex, needlework, cooking, reflecting on dreams, and a number of other interstitial practices. But from culture to culture, from region to region, versions of this distinction between 'first' and 'second' sleep would invariably appear. In some cultures, people were supposed to take the first sleep on their right side and the second on their left, giving rise to the expression that one had got out of bed 'on the wrong side'.

In a few hundred years, this basic biology had become undone. By the mid 1800s, references to the two sleeps were on the wane and consolidated sleep was increasingly becoming the norm. Ekirch at first linked this to the rise of artificial lighting, as gas and then electric lights were to replace the oil lamps that had appeared on city streets in the seventeenth century. These technological changes meant that not only could shops and businesses stay open later, but that a whole new culture of night-time could emerge. Historians have charted this extraordinary metamorphosis of city life, which would push back the boundary of the first and subsequently only sleep.

Artificial lighting opened up new possibilities, undermining the received associations of light and darkness, and both encouraged and facilitated later bedtimes. The century between 1730 and 1830 was the key time for changing bedtimes due to nocturnal activities. London had some 5,000 oil lamps in 1736 and 40,000 gas lamps by 1823, while Paris had a mere 200 gas lights in 1835 yet nearly 13,000 just four years later. The lamps were known not as 'street lights' but 'police lamps', showing the link between light and safety, yet the idea of surveillance worked in more than one sense. This was also the time that new habits became possible, such as staring into other people's homes after dark. This expansion of public and private lighting had massive effects on illumination: where a simple gas light could give about twelve times as much light as an oil lamp or candle, the electric bulbs that would appear towards the end of the nineteenth century were around a hundred times brighter.

If the early 'children of the night', as they were called by a contemporary writer, tended to be those of leisure and means, a far more widespread and radical process of change was at work beyond the gatherings and balls that the new culture accelerated. The less privileged would often be working later, as the new lighting technologies meant that shops and businesses could stay open well after dark. If sleep had for centuries acquired a spiritual meaning, as a time for purification and rest, these values were to be eroded. With the Industrial Revolution, sleep was becoming less a precious and perhaps personal space for renewal than a time that meant progressively . . . not being at work.

Ekirch added these social and economic dimensions to his account of the causes of the loss of biphasic sleep, so they were not limited to the expansion and refinement of urban lighting. Shifts in how work itself was understood, the rise of shift work and scheduling, new technologies and their impact on production processes, the concept of time management and notions of a work 'ethic' suited to industrial capitalism all worked together to create the move to the model of consolidated sleep. For Ekirch, it seemed clear that an original biological process was being warped by human social change.

When Ekirch learnt of the experiments of sleep researcher Thomas Wehr at the National Institute of Mental Health, it seemed he had found biological confirmation of his thesis. Wehr had isolated his subjects from the artificial light/dark partitions of modern life and found that many of them slept in not one but two segments. He had tried to create lighting conditions closer to the day–night cycle in winter, with his volunteers spending fourteen-hour blocks in a dark room after ten hours' exposure to light. Like Ekirch's pre-industrial populations, they would duly wake for periods of two to three hours after midnight before falling into a second sleep. The period of wakefulness or 'watching' thus seemed to occur 'naturally' with the loss of extended artificial light, the main culprit that Ekirch had identified in his historical studies. Consolidated sleep, it appeared, was a product of the Industrial Revolution, and biphasic sleep the original rhythm of the human body.

There is some controversy today around these claims. It is undeniable that a division of sleep into two phases was a standard part of human experience in many cultures until the nineteenth century, but whether the body reverts to it if deprived of artificial light is not so certain. If Wehr's experiments appeared to confirm it, other researchers have had more ambiguous results, although the sleep patterns they found instead have almost all tended towards interrupted periods of sleeping. Much of this research, however, rests on a fantasy, the idea that the way to find the natural state of the human body is through isolating it.

To discover the original, primitive rhythm of sleep, an individual is cut off from the social body. They are isolated in a cave, an underground bunker or a special sleep lab, while technologies monitor activity cycles, temperature, hormone levels, and so on. Although this may reveal some significant results about environmental cues to physiological processes, it doesn't tell us too much about 'natural' sleep given the fact that humans live next to or close to each other, and it is precisely this proximity that may have powerful effects, as we shall see, in shaping sleep.

Almost all of the main variables in sleep physiology are altered if an infant sleeps with its mother, ranging from neurochemical concentrations, to the amount of deep sleep, to respiratory behaviour. The experiments that seek to actively separate the sleeper are reminiscent of Louis II's isolation of babies from human language to see if their first words were in Hebrew or Latin. The mistake here is not to see language – and sleep – as involving social relations with others. Sleep, like language, may be something that we have to learn. Rather than simply sleeping, as children we are 'put' to sleep, and later, as adults, we have to 'put ourselves' to sleep in increasingly complex ways.

Switching Off

The story of our move from a natural biphasic sleep to one block of consolidated sleep chimes well with current nostalgia for an original organic world in which people once lived in harmony with nature. But things are not really so simple. Thompson's vision of a task-oriented agricultural society may be wish-fulfilment, and he certainly underestimated the presence of time-keeping practices in the early-modern world. In their careful study of timekeeping in late-medieval and early-modern England, Paul Glennie and Nigel Thrift show how daily life was filled with temporal markers well before the industrial period began. Religious houses, schools, markets, guilds and sporting events all involved marking times of day, as did the expanding postal and transportation networks. Coach hire, indeed, was priced by duration rather than by distance.

Similarly, the idea of an agricultural society governed purely by the cycle of day and night is questionable. Such societies, after all, do not set their clocks simply by sunrise and sunset, and workers may well wake at 3 a.m. in order to finish harvesting by the late morning. Some crops, indeed, cannot be easily processed after midday, when their leaves become sticky and unmanageable, just as others cannot be harvested at sunrise due to the presence of dew. When we imagine that the happy agricultural worker would be woken at sunrise by the cock's crow, work in the fields, and then enjoy a refreshing sleep, we should remember that cocks crow several times during the night, marking different dawns, and that at the day's close, many other forms of work would be necessary, from treating crops and making repairs, to spinning, preparing food and cleaning. Hundreds of years before artificial lighting, work would continue well after sunset.

This is not to downplay the effects of industrialisation, artificial lighting and the new work ethics of early capitalism – which no doubt had effects on how people experienced time – but simply to question the idea of an earlier agricultural harmony governed by the cycle of day and night. The critic Jonathan Crary has the lovely formula that capitalism is not compatible with the axial rotation of the earth, but then neither was pre-capitalism. The day–night cycle was perhaps more important then than it was later in some parts of the world, but human beings have always been disconnected from their habitats, introducing their own artificial metrics, hierarchies and prohibitions to govern their relation with their surroundings. Clock time and timekeeping practices have never been entirely in synch with day–night cycles, as we see from even the most basic facts of seasonal variation.

As time gradually became standardised, the fact that a true twenty-four-hour day occurs only four times a year attracted little attention. The earth's elliptical orbit, its changing speed as it travels around the sun and the fact that it moves closer to the sun at certain times of the year lost out to the homogeneity of the mechanical clock. Although timekeeping practices have a long history, and clocks themselves pre-date the Industrial Revolution, it was arguably the nineteenth century's communications systems of telegraphy and the railroads that established the dominion of the new timekeeping with their promise of ever-swifter connectivity.

This is why we speak of modern 'times': it meant that local solar times were replaced by time zones and national mean times. In solar time, noon was marked by the sun crossing the meridian, and so different places had different times depending on their longitudinal position. By the mid 1870s, about seventy-five railway times were in use in the US, with more than one often marked within the same city. Parallel times were very common, with court and railroad clocks set to different times on the same street. German officials considered giving station clocks two hands, one for local time and one for railway time, a practice that took place in France but with two clocks, one inside and one outside the station, while some even had a third clock set to Paris time.

The car manufacturer Henry Ford described how when he was just a poor handyman repairing jewellery and watches, he already had the idea of making a timepiece with two dials: one for local 'sun time' and the other for 'standard railroad time', as if geographical separation had to be negated in order for business to progress. This canny invention must have seemed like a novelty at the time – 'it was quite a curiosity in the neighbourhood', says Ford – yet today, rather than being on the wrist, it is as if the two clocks are internalised. Our productivity must satisfy multiple masters, and this means that the clock never stops. As Crary points out, we have moved beyond the old division between on and off: in today's marketplace, and indeed, in our personal

lives, there is no longer any real state of rest, and pa...
must be artificially generated – and paid for.

—

With industrialisation and new frameworks to organise
and regiment workers' lives, sleep came to occupy a
spectrum between, on the one hand, the minimum necessary to allow continued production of goods, and on
the other, a principle of sacrifice for the greater good.
For many employers and employees, sleep should be
given up to ensure a proper work ethic. The old British
proverb, popularised by Benjamin Franklin, 'Early to
bed and early to rise', could be compared with the Chinese aphorism, 'Late to bed and early to rise'. And how
early and late were measured would depend less on the
cycle of day and night and more on the effects of the
twenty-four-hour clock, which differs from solar time.
This is nowhere more apparent than in contemporary
China, which, despite its massive size, in 1949 abolished
all its previous five time zones in favour of one standard
Chinese time. The unique Beijing Time was a metaphor
of national unity, showing how time can serve a political
purpose.

Individual lives are of course the casualties here.
When we in the West contact a service provider in the
evening and find ourselves speaking to someone in India
or Asia, we may make the assumption that the reason
the call is being outsourced is that our evening is their
morning. The outsourcing makes sense in terms of
global time differences. Yet in many cases, the person on
the other end of the phone is in fact a night-shift worker,
staying up to serve a more dominant economy and earn

the meagre wage that they are paid there. Local economies are aligned with more powerful foreign ones, with the body's need for sleep deemed secondary in this imbalance. Some sleep clinics even outsource in this way, sending data abroad despite being well aware of the negative effects of shift work.

We can see this continuous profit-making process reflected nicely in the straplines of the two famous *Wall Street* films. In 1987, the posters declared: 'Every dream has a price', indicating the moral poverty that accompanied financial avarice. In the 2014 sequel, the strapline read: 'Money never sleeps', moving the emphasis away from any moral question to a simple affirmation of the reality of the market. If sleep is supposed to take up roughly a third of one's life, money takes up all of it. And it is this colonisation of both the body and time that capitalism necessarily involves.

If money never sleeps, the breaks and interruptions of everyday life become either dispensed with or commodified in themselves. A coffee, a chocolate bar or – until recently – a cigarette are equated with the time spent enjoying them. This time must be paid for, but that does not just mean buying the product in question, since we also now fill this time with work, checking our phones and computers and in general multitasking. Any real pause seems improbable, and this erosion of the structure of our day is reflected not simply in the loss of biphasic sleep but in the gradual disappearance of the traditional daytime nap.

From the Spanish siesta to the Japanese *inemuri*, anthropologists and sociologists have documented in some detail how these practices are vanishing. In Spain, the government decided in 2006 to ban workplace napping in civil service and public offices, while in Japan, the daytime sleep taken in locations as disparate as meetings and parties is increasingly frowned on, and in many places no longer permitted. Lunchtime napping in China, which was made part of the constitution in 1950, is also subject to prohibitions, with break time reduced dramatically from three hours to just one. The underlying logic here is of course the market, as human time is profit, and napping will detract from productivity and efficiency. Just as money never sleeps, so too its human servants are deprived of the pauses and breaks that once formed part of daily life.

Interestingly, although sleep hygienists have often pointed out that productivity can be increased by workplace napping, the many attempts to introduce this practice in the West have not been so successful. Companies like Pepsi, IBM and Pizza Hut have all run courses on how to take a fifteen-minute power nap, and dedicated spaces such as workplace sleep pods and special sleep areas, with dim lights and leafy plants, have been experimented with. Popular books with titles like *Sleep for Success* and *The Art of Napping at Work* extol the benefits of the workplace nap, and have predicted that it will become part of the working day. Despite the well-being rhetoric, however, many of these ventures have failed, and companies formed to sell sleeping spaces to large corporations have gone out of business. It is difficult, after all, not only to change established sleeping habits, but also to exorcise the relentless imperatives that fill the average working day. The imperative to now take a nap can just seem like one more of them. The irony here is that both sleep and the cancellation of sleep serve the same master: economic productivity.

———

There is a clear and disturbing conflict of messages here. On the one hand, we inhabit an unsleeping world of commerce and information, and on the other, we are increasingly told to get the right number of hours of good uninterrupted sleep. The two, of course, are not compatible, and it is in the space opened up by these contradictory imperatives that a lot of money can be made. Professionals can offer to reprogramme your sleep, and pharmaceutical companies can sell you pills to do it. Rather than recognising the impossible reconciliation of imperatives, it becomes the very principle for marketisation.

Yet how can we retreat to what is supposed to be the old rhythm of sleep and wakefulness if we are expected to be in a perpetual state of arousal? Phones, laptops and our other electronic devices continue to clock up demands as we sleep, and there are now several new apps that offer to protect us: they promise to make us unavailable, bracketing off messages and demands. We have to use our phones and computers, then, to protect us from our phones and computers. Which means of course remembering to set the app, to check it, to monitor it as it supposedly monitors us.

It is instructive to note here how in the bedtime classic *Goodnight Moon* – published in 1947 and still a favourite today – each object in the bunny's home is named and then bidden farewell: a telephone, a red balloon, a toy house, a young mouse, two kittens and a pair of mittens . . . The symmetry of naming every element and then saying goodnight to it is no doubt restful, yet curiously the very first object to be named in the inventory is the only one that does not receive a goodnight: the telephone.

This conduit to external demands is magnified in the smartphones and tablets that now lie on our bedside tables, opening us up not only to calls, but to texts, emails and all manner of social media communications and feeds. The surveys that seem to belie this are perhaps symptomatic in their own way. When questioned about whether they feel more interpellated by work demands via their computers and smartphones after working hours have officially finished, many people report that this is not the case and that they are perfectly able to switch off. Yet this surely indicates a second feature of our times, the pressure to pretend that everything is okay, something that contrasts quite radically with earlier periods in the twentieth century, when it was permissible and even expected to show that things were not okay.

In his brilliant exposition of 'looping', Erving Goffman differentiated everyday social space and that of 'total institutions' such as prisons and asylums. In ordinary working life, he argued, we are able to register affronts to our sense of self through face-saving reactive expressions: sullenness, failure to defer, lack of enthusiasm, negative asides, scowling, expressions of irony, and so on. But in total institutions, the agencies that create these defensive responses then take them as the next target of attack. The inmate cannot establish any distance between his mortifying situation and himself, as the ways in which he would do this now become further reasons for being punished. But crucially, beyond the question of a concrete punishment, the scowl or the sarcastic comment is taken to define the individual rather than the individual's response to their dreadful situation.

As Goffman puts it, the signs of an individual's disaffiliation are now read as signs of their affiliation. If the inmate of an asylum finds him- or herself in seclusion, naked and with no visible means of expression, tearing up a mattress or writing with faeces on the cell wall are not seen as legitimate procedures but simply as further evidence that the person requires incarceration. The less able the person is to make themselves heard, the more their efforts will be used to define them as warranting their punishment. Staff, indeed, are often too stretched to record anything other than acts of disobedience.

Today we are surely witnessing an expansion of what Goffman saw as a characteristic of the prison and the asylum to all social spaces, where negativity is seen as a sign of pathology. Through the process of looping, expressions of withdrawal or discontent – in other words, legitimate reactions to one's situation – become collapsed back into the situation itself. We have to be passionate and focused on all our projects and endeavours, feigning enthusiasm for mundane, stupid tasks and camaraderie for detested colleagues and co-workers. To cap all of this is the continuous pressure to both self-evaluate and be evaluated. And isn't this exactly what so many insomniacs describe, that as they lie in bed, what haunts them is the question: how have I done today?

Avoiding Complexity

It is tempting to guess that the erosion of the spaces that Goffman describes, where we are able to mark a distance from the demands made upon us, will result in the search for another place in which to do so, perhaps the very border between waking and sleeping. As we lie awake, all the scowls, withdrawals and asides we neglected to make can be imagined, together with the acts of revenge and reprisal required to preserve our dignity. As the writer Chloe Aridjis puts it, it is now that the 'thoughts that emitted a quiet glow during the day become radioactive'. But even in the privacy of our beds, the total institution is still there. As one of my patients described it, 'I'm just lying there for hours, going over the day again and again, asking myself what have I achieved, again and again and again.' And of course this question of what has been achieved swiftly becomes the question: what did I do wrong today?

Nearly all interactions, indeed, are now accompanied by the request for feedback, as if human behaviour is essentially something that can be improved and worked on. We often hear it said that artificial intelligence poses a grave problem here, as machines risk becoming more and more like us, and that hence new dangers and threats will emerge. But isn't it the other way round? When one looks at the AI research of the late 1940s and 50s, everyone is trying to find a way for machines to be able not simply to perform an operation but then, as the crucial step, to ask: how have I done? This feedback will then have to be incorporated into their subsequent performance. Yet what was then seen as an ideal function of a machine has now become the baseline for ordinary human life.

Whereas traditional machines dealt with the metabolism of engines – that is, the transformation of one form of energy into another – the so-called servomechanisms developed during the Second World War aimed to simulate goal-directed behaviour. A comparison between their own performance and a prescribed state would itself become an input, known as a feedback loop. The servosystem would thus be responding not only to the external world but to its own response to the external world. This was very useful for target-seeking missiles, but what it meant was effectively a progressive assimilation not of machines to us but of us to machines.

The vocabulary of artificial machine technology and AI, such as 'feedback', shifted from machines to humans, so that we now have to embody the very procedures that they were supposed to be mimicking. In this strange transposition, it is the humans and not just the machines that spend their lives going round asking: how have I performed? How can I be better? What are my strengths and weaknesses? These were exactly the questions that the early servosystems were supposed to ask themselves. And like these machines and their more sophisticated descendants, we are now always 'on', with less and less possibility to revert to a world in which 'on/off' has any meaning.

Even on television variety shows, we no longer just

watch singers, dancers and entertainers, but the performers plus a jury who sit there in judgement of them. In effect, what we are watching is evaluation as such, with the question 'How have I performed?' turned into entertainment, yet the pain and disappointment of those involved is visible behind the forced smiles. We aren't simply watching someone sing, but sing and then be judged. Shows like *The Apprentice* recapitulate this, with the real fascination focused less on how tasks are performed than on the harshness and brutality with which they are evaluated. Like the machines, it is no longer a question of just doing things but of doing them and then asking 'Could I have done better?'

Curiously, the winners of such shows often end up appearing on a second and then a third reality show, rather than settling in to the job or career that the first one had promised them. If you win *The Apprentice*, you can go on to *Celebrity Big Brother*, and then, if you're lucky, to *Dancing on Ice*. As they are passed round from show to show, it is as if the new profession of these figures is to be continually visible and monitored, evaluated at all times by new judges and audiences. Their career consists of little more than being assessed in public.

These shows are also symptoms of the decline of the traditional figures of authority in modern life. Social theorists describe how father figures of all sorts are reduced from Jehovah-type lawgivers to powerless clowns, and this means that the wish to resurrect them is often strong. As both legal and social forces restrict – or try to restrict – the unchecked exercise of patriarchal power, a void is created that, rather than becoming the space for a new parity, may favour the re-establishment of an imbalance. As the authority figure becomes increasingly subject to the law, unable to wield power without proper regulation and external sanction, so he reappears in the TV show as entertainment, humiliating and demeaning contestants, following his own caprice with little regard for anyone's well-being or dignity. While irrational authority is decried in the media, this is what people choose to watch, a sort of return of the repressed in the guise of a variety show.

The bizarre twist to this logic was evident in the US election of Donald Trump. This was someone who owed a great deal of his popularity to a TV show, *The Apprentice*, in which he filled precisely this role of authority and caprice transformed into entertainment. Yet when he then went on to become president, for many it made no sense at all: the strange sense of unreality felt by millions of Americans testified to the reversal of a psychical process. This was very different to the election of Ronald Reagan, for example, an actor who became president. People could find this laughable or distasteful, but not genuinely uncanny, as was the case with Trump, who took on the very role for which his public persona in *The Apprentice* had been a sort of symptomatic compensation.

Visions of the future that show a seamless fit between human life and technology are both correct and incorrect here. There is no doubt that an ever-increasing incursion of AI into everyday life and human services will take place, and there is also no doubt that this will not fit, that there will be a fracture or 'basic fault' between us and machines. A doctor can never really be replaced by AI, for example, but this will not stop investment in the replacement of many medical services from happening. But the key here is to recognise that what this means is not some sort of moment of enlightenment when we realise what machines can and can't do but, on the contrary, an ever-increasing pressure on us to be like machines. If we aren't happy with an AI doctor, this will mean that we, and not the AI doctor, need to change. We will have to become more and more like whatever it is that an AI doctor can treat.

＊

We can see many of these changes reflected in the literature on sleep. It is quite striking to compare the scientific and popular publications of the 1960s and 70s with those of today. The earlier studies seem sober and humane, recognising the difficulties of life, whereas much of the new sleep science assumes that we inhabit some sort of fantasy world in which people can live rich, full and satisfied lives once they nail their sleep problem, usually identified with purely external factors that can be modified through behavioural change.

When I buy my morning coffee, I always ask the baristas if they have woken up happy and refreshed, looking forward to the day ahead. We all laugh, just because the idea is so absurd, and yet the supposition of this kind of fulfilled life underlies much of contemporary sleep hygiene. Where Ernest Hartmann's seminal 1978 book, *The Sleeping Pill*, tells us on its first page that 'To a certain extent life *is* pain and sorrow', by 2017 Matthew Walker's *Why We Sleep* sings the praises of man as a kind of champion among animals, superior to all other beasts, whose sleep gives him unique powers of rationality and creativity. Rapid eye movement sleep – on which more later – helped man gain his 'rapid evolution-ary rise to power' and constitute a 'globally dominant social superclass'. 'Sleep', says Walker, 'recalibrates our emotional brain circuits, allowing us to navigate next-day social and psychological challenges with cool-headed composure' so that we attain a 'level-headed ability to read the social world around us'.

Whereas in Gay Luce and Julius Segal's bestselling 1969 book, *Insomnia*, the opening sentence reads: 'There is only one sure way to escape insomnia . . . not to be born', in the more recent sleep literature, there is no place for human fracture and dislocation. We can read today that sleep helped us to become 'emotionally astute, stable, highly bonded and intensely social com-munities of humans', a diagnosis that does not fit what I see on the news every day or learn from world history. The new pressures to sell ideas and to paper over the realities of human life, together with the looping effect described by Goffman, mean that we are coerced into a well-being-speak, constantly demonstrating positivity and enthusiasm. If you don't have a smile on your face, there must be something wrong with you, and the ubi-quity of emojis in everyday life is testimony to this. The complexity of real emotions has become so unaccept-able today that these cartoon caricatures have literally taken their place, not only in texting and emails but even in many of the disciplines that claim to be science.

Whereas in the 1920s and 30s, naive Darwinian views of emotion were deconstructed and shown to be hopelessly inadequate, today these very same views are actually used as templates in scientific experiments. The old nineteenth-century theory was that there were between six and nine basic emotions, which correlated with specific physiological expressions that could be found in any culture. Anger, joy and disgust were just real things, revealed unambiguously through the human face. Anthropologists and psychiatrists pointed out, on the contrary, that expressions formed part of communicative exchanges with others, and hence were socially determined and linked to expectations and assumptions specific to the human group in question. To isolate the person and then film their facial expressions won't reveal any deeper truth, as we all internalise the social systems that we grow up within. We wear masks even when we are on our own.

A patient in a brain scanner is shown a picture of a smiling or an angry face, and the resultant trace of blood oxygenation taken to represent the state of happiness or rage. The cues can be more sophisticated – images or words that have been deemed disturbing or pleasant – but the structure is more or less the same. Facial expression is understood here as identical with a set number of innate emotions linked to our evolutionary heritage. What people feel is not linked to the particularity of their own history but to certain 'objective' elements that are taken to embody goodness or badness. This is no different from the world of emojis, where complex human emotions are taken to be discrete particles that can be neatly segregated. The emoji says, 'This is how I feel', but real life, not to mention world literature and probably the whole of human culture, shows, on the contrary, that emotions cannot be compartmentalised like this and that they may metamorphose and blur into each other.

Just as fear and desire can oscillate and become the

poles of an equation, so attraction and disgust can easily become equal. 'Sadness and rage', an analysand says, 'are the same thing for me, there's no difference.' 'Fear', says another, 'becomes sexual desire.' 'I feel both devastated and liberated,' says another on the death of a parent. So which emoji should she use? Anthropologists have long shown how emotions are part of social behaviour, both experienced and made meaningful by our interactions and relationships with others, and organised by cultural rules of expression. Olympic gold medallists, as the historian of affect Ruth Leys points out, produce many facial expressions during the medal ceremony but only smile when interacting with the audience and officials, showing that the smile is not a natural pre-programmed response indexing an underlying emotion but something that is determined by social interaction.

Why this return to notions that have long been refuted? For Leys, it resonates with the modern imperative to read the person through bodily signs, as if a facial expression is like a printout of a discrete internal state. Properly trained observers can then access a person's inner truth through an act of reading, as if this were independent of any ideology or meaning. Emotions themselves become products that can be localised and distinguished the one from the other, commodities that require precise differentiation and valuation. In the early 1990s, I was teaching at a university in Paris when Disneyland was just about to open there. The park contacted us to offer part-time jobs to students, whose brief was essentially to wander round smiling and greeting visitors. If this happy face was paid for, today it is simply expected of all of us. What was once seen as a piece of theatre to be remunerated is now just the baseline of almost all human operations.

As market-based societies increasingly practised an atomisation of the social group, so that 'citizens' became 'individuals' who were seen as isolated economic units in competition with each other for goods and services, the academic psychology of the twentieth and now the twenty-first century provided an underpinning. The human subject was less a part of a social group with collective responsibilities and duties than an autonomous agent with rights, defined by one-dimensional instrumental goals: the pursuit of wealth, happiness, success and health. Whereas for centuries the human psyche had been characterised by conflict – between reason and emotion, between the will and education, between the ego and the unconscious – it is as if now the soul is conflict-free, just striving for one simple and unambiguous goal.

Again, compare the sleep literature of the 1960s with that of today. Luce and Segal write that the person who lies awake at night is no different from the person who struggled through the day, 'the same personality who loved and hated, laughed or cried, and swerved from peace to anxiety'. But in the universe of many contemporary sleep hygienists, there is no contradiction. Life, we can read, is governed by two simple rules that dictate most of human and animal behaviour: 'staying away from something that would feel bad, or trying to accomplish something that would feel good'. This is 'science' in the twenty-first century. The emotions that drive this law, we are told, are what make us try again when we fail, keep us safe from potential harm, urge us to accomplish rewarding and beneficial outcomes, and compel us to cultivate social and romantic relationships.

In this strange one-dimensional world, it seems as if just about the only place where anyone can still recognise that we might strive for contradictory things – both success and failure, both wealth and poverty, both health and sickness – is in *Star Wars*. The franchise trades on the old childhood idea that there is something special in all of us just waiting to be recognised, glossed here as the 'Force' that we can discover within ourselves. But crucially, the narratives revolve around those powerful moments when a character finds themself torn between contradictory allegiances, between this 'Force' and the 'Dark Side', as if the matter is never finally settled and the very core of our being consists in this dreadful battle between opposing tendencies.

In the case we discussed earlier, the wish to sleep conflicted with the wish to have an insomnia diagnosed and acknowledged. By focusing only on one of these currents, we risk neglecting the other and thus losing the essence of the person's difficulties. And with that, we also lose the possibility of helping them to move forward. Human beings are divided in many ways, and what appears as paradox or contradiction is ignored at our cost. Not sleeping can be a torment, but it may also fulfil a function, materialising a punishment – as we shall see – or acting as an appeal for some other form of pain to be recognised.

What is Sleep?

If artificial lighting, changes linked to capitalism and new work ethics altered the way that sleep was construed, by the later part of the nineteenth century a two-part biphasic sleep was seen as problematic. Where for centuries, waking up in the night was not the occasion for worry or alarm but simply part of the course of things, it had now become pathologised as an anomaly. Both medical textbooks and lay self-help books warned of the dangers of middle-of-the-night waking, and remedies and medicines were widely advertised.

When the psychoanalyst Frances Deri received a young medical student in the early 1930s who complained of his lack of concentration when studying, there was no initial discussion of any sleep issues. After several months, he casually remarked, 'My wake-hour's from two to three', as if he took it for granted that everyone had a 'wake-hour'. When Deri queried this, he 'began to deliver a sort of lecture about the fact that everybody, regardless of whether he was a good sleeper or a bad one, had one definite hour of the night during which he did not sleep'. He would himself turn in at around ten or eleven, sleep soundly until two, then wake for around an hour, with no resentment or effort to return to sleep, before drifting off again until seven. Deri comments: 'It was not very easy to convince him of the symptomatic character of his wake-hour.'

What is so remarkable about the vignette is that the patient's description of his nocturnal rhythm is exactly what historians and anthropologists describe as the authentic structure of human sleep. The only problem is that it was a few decades past its societal sell-by date. The analyst tries to make him recognise that his sleep pattern is abnormal, a symptom that requires treatment, yet all he is doing is following the biphasic sleep pattern of his ancestors. What would have attracted no attention at all perhaps some sixty years earlier had now, by the 1930s, become a sign of illness.

We see here how our expectations of what sleep ought to be will shape what we consider to be abnormal or pathological. Perhaps Deri's patient was simply following an age-old pattern of human sleep, but as consolidated sleep became the new norm, biphasic sleep became the problem. Even in a time where consolidated sleep is taken by many to be its natural state, new pathologies are generated each time the latest opinion is turned into a fact about sleep: the experts may say eight hours at one moment and seven at another, just as some of the breathing particularities of sleep may seem peripheral at one moment and signs of disease at another.

Echoing these changes, the term 'insomnia' began to appear in late nineteenth-century dictionaries with a medical meaning beyond the general sense of sleeplessness that it held previously, and the back pages of newspapers and periodicals were filled with offers for products that would deliver sleep. Powders, ointments, potions and plasters all promised a peaceful night. Whereas before the mid to late 1800s, difficulties in falling asleep had been more commonly reported, it was now waking up during the night that was considered the central problem. Ekirch argues that during these years there was a progressive confusion of the inability to fall asleep with this new emphasis on the inability to remain asleep, which was often linked in both medical and lay texts with the pressures of modern living.

In the late 1860s, a New York businessman could complain of how 'reports of the principal markets are published every day, and our customers are continually posted by telegram'. He was thus 'kept in continual excitement, without time for quiet or rest', returning home 'perhaps after a long day of hard work and excitement, to a late dinner, trying amid the family circle to forget business when he is interrupted by a telegram from London'. 'Sleeplessness', wrote another commentator on insomnia in the 1880s, 'has been much of late' attributed to 'the practical annihilation of time and space by our telegraphs and railroads, the compressing thereby of the labors of months into hours or even minutes, the terrific competition in all kinds of business thereby made possible and inevitable, the intense mental activity engendered in the mad race for fame and wealth, where the nervous and mental force of man is measured against steam and lightning'.

An article on 'Sleeplessness' in the *British Medical Journal* in 1894 could state that 'The hurry and excitement of modern life is quite correctly held to be responsible for much of the insomnia of which we hear.' In terms strikingly similar to those used today, the 'chronic terror' of insomnia was linked to the new technologies that collapsed space and time. If the very idea of a single night's unbroken sleep was in many ways a product of the

Industrial Revolution, then the idea of what breaks our sleep and what can remedy this was also shaped by social change. And certainly, by the early twenty-first century, a shift in how we perceive sleep problems has been firmly established. If there is still an acknowledgement that 'worry' and 'stress' are causes of insomnia, lack of sleep is now being used to explain these very anxieties. As more and more human difficulties are seen through the lens of sleep disorders, the damage they cause seems limitless. Where depressive states were once linked to grief or repressed rage, and then to a chemical imbalance in the brain, now they are often ascribed to a lack of sleep.

Yet if what we expect from sleep generates the way we conceive of and categorise sleep disorders, is everything here relative? Is there not some real and immutable number of hours that we need or does it depend purely on cultural imperatives? To argue that sleep is either biological or social is to miss the point, since the two cannot be distinguished in any absolute sense here. Although these imperatives have clearly changed over the years, it is also a fact that people have always suffered from lack of sleep, even if how this suffering was displayed and understood has changed over time.

When historians of sleep point to the burgeoning of sleep pathology during the nineteenth century and link this to the development of factory labour, artificial lighting and the modern market, this may well be true, but at the same time the focus on medical publications draws attention away from a much older tradition, which testifies to the continual problems people experienced at night-time. If we turn not to medical texts but to cookbooks, we see that for centuries recipes have been proffered that enable sleep or calm night-time anxiety. Interspersed with the household recipes, there would invariably be those 'To cause one to sleep'.

—

But what is sleep here? The writer Georgie Byng points out that so many sleep therapies involve focusing on an inert, restful image or relaxation process, as if 'we need to trick or fool ourselves into sleep'. A placid blue sea or a green field are summoned in order to extinguish the thoughts that keep us awake, or are simply what wakefulness consists of. The need for a certain mental gymnastics to access sleep suggests that it is hardly a natural state, and that if we have to cheat ourselves to procure it, there is even an incompatibility between sleep and the self.

Likewise, once we have it, it can so easily disappear. Perhaps surprisingly, it is only relatively recently that sleep researchers claim to have come up with an answer as to why we sleep. Although there have always been plenty of theories, biology texts from the late nineteenth to the late twentieth century could still claim that sleep remained a mystery. If a process like breathing brooks a relatively simple explanation – to inhale oxygen and exhale carbon dioxide – this is not the case for sleep. If its function is purely physiological, what exactly does it do? And if also psychological, what is its purpose?

It might seem obvious that sleep is what allows the organism to recharge, like a battery. It would be a natural state that follows human activity, brought on by fatigue or exhaustion. Yet such explanations have been eschewed by almost everyone who has studied sleep seriously. Those who remain inactive may sleep exactly the same amount or even longer than those who do athletics all day, so the link between activity and sleep is not evident. The Swiss psychologist Édouard Claparède, for example, argued that sleep was in fact a defence against fatigue, not a result of it, and various experiments have shown that people may actually have difficulty in falling asleep if they are kept awake for a long period.

If it was just exhaustion that allowed sleep, likewise, would there be so much insomnia? As for the battery model, the idea that we need to re-energise or conserve precious energy is complicated by the fact that, as we shall see, we are actually very active during the night, and the amount of energy we save by a good night's sleep is equivalent only to roughly one glass of wine (80 to 130 calories). Although our metabolism may slow down, and our temperature, heart rate and pulse drop, the effect on the conservation of energy is not as dramatic as we might have expected. Even the energy requirement of the brain is hardly affected: cerebral oxygen consumption drops only by 2.8 per cent.

Yet no one really doubts here that sleep is essential. Circadian and other rhythmic processes clearly push us towards sleep, as do the build-up and depletion of certain chemicals in the body. To find an explanation, a strategy of sleep deprivation has often been used: if you can figure out what happens when a human being – or more often, a cat or a rat – is deprived of sleep, then it will shed light on what the functions of sleep might be. Again, this has generated some fascinating research, with some very relevant medical implications, but its broader logic is open to question: if someone starts to hallucinate, say, or dies after being sleep-deprived, does it follow that the purpose of sleep is to stop us hallucinating or dying? Or, if it is true that sleep deprivation weakens our ability to kill, that sleep is there to allow us to take lives?

On the other hand, to learn that immune functioning and tissue repair is accentuated during sleep – and that sleep deprivation will thus compromise how the body wards off illness – may seem more persuasive as a teleology. But why sleep rather than rest here? What kind of a condition is sleep and what is supposed to actually happen within it? The usual story here is that for centuries sleep was considered a passive state, until the development in the late 1920s of human electroencephalography (EEG), which allowed a study of the brain's electrical activity during sleep, and in the early 1950s of rapid eye movement sleep (REM), considered the real game-changer in sleep science.

Electrodes placed on the scalp recorded the fluctuations of electrical potentials, indicative of activity of local areas of the brain. The measurement of these potentials over a defined period of time created the image of 'brain waves', which showed considerable variation during the night-time hours. It seemed clear that the brain was immensely busy at night, and that the EEG readings of REM sleep resembled bizarrely those of the waking state. Many researchers even suggested that REM periods should not be called 'sleep' at all, and a variety of different names were proposed: paradoxical sleep, archi sleep, rapid sleep, activated sleep and dreaming sleep.

In the REM periods, the EEG reading indicated that the subject was in some sense awake, though they were clearly asleep. Their eyes were closed, their body seemed more or less immobile, and they were unresponsive to stimuli. Eugene Aserinsky, working under Nathaniel Kleitman at the University of Chicago, called these the 'Rapid Eye Movement periods', with the emphasis on the period. He had favoured 'Jerky Eye Movement', as he was struck by their jerkiness and they were less rapid than eye movements in waking life, but decided against this due to the association of 'jerk' with masturbation.

It was thus no longer a question of sleep and wakefulness, but of sleep, wakefulness and REM sleep, a transitional state between waking and sleeping that seemed to many researchers to be much closer to waking than to sleep. Non-REM sleep (NREM) was itself divided into five, then four and more recently three different phases, and the relations between these states was and continues to be explored. When we are awake, we tend to have low-amplitude but high-frequency waves, the latter taken to indicate how awake or vigilant we are. As we become tired, the higher frequencies fade, and we find alpha rhythms, slower waves characteristic of the drowsy state.

The amplitude of the waves will now increase, and we pass from the alpha rhythm of relaxed waking to Stage 1 NREM. This is usually taken to be a transitional stage, with some researchers once requiring the absence of alpha rhythms but most accepting that there should be less than 50 per cent alpha activity, a decision made more complex by the fact that, according to sleep researcher Ian Oswald, about 10 per cent of the population do not display alpha rhythms in the first place. Slower-frequency theta waves are present – sometimes linked to repetitive, mind-numbing tasks – and it is during this phase that we can experience sharp jerks, which sometimes wake us up, and which can be the source of some perplexity. If we do wake in this sleep stage, we may also be struck by vivid visual and acoustic images called hypnagogic phenomena, on which more later.

The Stage 2 NREM that follows takes up 45 to 50 per cent of total sleep time, and is characterised by low-amplitude waves, with ripples of much faster activity called spindling, and K-complexes, small, sharp waves that can precipitate awakening and a return to alpha rhythm. A K-complex can appear after stimulation of any sense modality, yet can be habituated, so a sound that initially causes a K-complex will have no effect after being repeated a few times. The fact that a K-complex can be generated by hearing one's name during sleep suggests that it is a partial arousal that responds to meaningful stimuli, although many researchers believe that it serves, on the contrary, to suppress acoustic and other disturbances and hence allows uninterrupted sleep.

Stages 3 and 4 are known as deep or slow-wave sleep, and it is interesting to see how they have been cropped down to only one stage in recent protocols. Whether this reduction is a progress or a way of avoiding problems that need to be explained is an open question. Stages 3 and 4 are made up of slow delta waves with some spindling, with delta waves at more than 50 per cent in Stage 4 and between 20 and 50 per cent in Stage 3. Stage 4 was originally defined as a very brief period of the deepest sleep, with little spindling and no K-complexes.

After these NREM stages have been run through, there is a return to Stage 2 prior to the REM period that follows, which is characterised by bursts of rapid eye movement, loss of muscle tone, a low-amplitude EEG that resembles waking, and irregular breathing and heart rate. This can last from a few minutes to half an hour or more, taking up progressively more time in the latter part of the night, and making up between 20 and 25 per cent of the night's sleep, although for newborns it takes up around 50 per cent. It can be interrupted by Stage 2 NREM, and, interestingly, a certain time has to elapse between one REM period and another. The cycle will then begin again, with average times for the whole run from Stage 1 to the end of the REM period taking between ninety and a hundred minutes, and with maybe thirty transitions between stages during an average seven-hour sleep.

After the first REM period, NREM Stage 1 will appear briefly, followed by Stage 2, but during the latter part of the night the presence of Stages 3 and 4 is significantly diminished. These times of deep slow-wave sleep occur mostly in the first part of the night, and it is a question why they should make such a limited appearance. Those who sleep for a block of between six and eight hours will have around four or five of the NREM–REM cycles each night, with the first REM period usually being very short, to be followed by a spell of slow-wave sleep. The next REM will be longer, and the cycles here tend to follow the ninety-minute rhythm.

The cycle length in newborns is shorter, averaging sixty minutes and increasing to around seventy-five by two years, although it is doubtful that the earliest REM is really like the REM of older children and adults. It is usually termed 'active sleep' or 'precursor REM', and is filled with twitches, smiles, grimaces, sucking motions and eye and limb movements. Their 'quiet sleep', in contrast, has less movement and eye activity, and more even breathing, with slower EEG, although readings here are often less helpful than direct observation. The other fascinating detail is that babies can enter sleep through precursor REM, whereas as they grow, this is no longer possible and NREM marks the entry into sleep. Developmentally, NREM appears to be a later stage than REM, established generally between three and five months.

REM sleep was characterised not only by eye movement but by bodily motility and less regular heart and respiratory rates. A link with dreams seemed obvious, as when woken from REM sleep there was a very high rate of dream recall compared with awakenings from NREM. This would generate a lot of excitement, and by the mid 1960s, dream research received what was considered then to be a staggering 5 per cent of the budget of the National Institute of Mental Health. Researchers asked the question of what biological and psychological function dreaming might have, and numerous experiments proved that stimuli such as noise and light could be registered during sleep, even if the person had no conscious memory of them. Blood pressure could rise dramatically with external noise even if the person continued to sleep through, with no awareness of what was happening.

These observations about sleep meant that it could no longer be considered a passive withdrawal from the world, which would follow automatically when we drew the curtains and turned off the TV. Horace Magoun and Giuseppe Moruzzi's work in the late 1940s on the active inhibition of the reticular formation during sleep was taken to confirm this idea of nocturnal activity. This part of the brain stem has branches – 'collaterals' – from sensory pathways together with fibres from higher brain centres, and, by adding its own activity, could influence changes in waking and sleeping behaviour independently of outside stimuli. The brain was thus very busy in controlling and generating both sleep and awakening

But perhaps the crucial discovery here was not that sleep had phases with different EEG tracings – which had been known for a long time – but that there was a real periodicity involved. In his earliest work, Aserinsky found that in each hourly motility cycle of infants there was a period of about twenty minutes when eye movements were greatly reduced. He would then try to correlate this with the REM periods in adults, which had a similar duration and also reduced muscle tension. Although he never managed to explain why this strange echo occurred, he showed how REM cycles occurred at specific points during the night. It was the periodicity that mattered.

Working throughout the night, Aserinsky's eye movement recording papers would stretch to up to half a mile long. The REM would only appear after the other sleep stages had been run through, and then emerge roughly every ninety minutes during the night. This was a stage of sleep that appeared periodically in a near-cyclic way, with EEG characteristics that differed from both waking and sleeping. There was – and still is – a real question here as to why the sequencing of NREM and REM occurred as it did. What was the function of these different stages? And what place did dreaming have within them?

———

Like most stories of scientific discovery, this one proves to be more complex. The idea that sleep was a highly active state was well known in the nineteenth century, particularly to European sleep researchers, and rapid eye movement was hardly a revelation. Dement says that the observation of rapid eye movements during sleep in the early 1950s was 'the breakthrough, the discovery that changed the course of sleep research', yet it was a phenomenon that had been described centuries previously and studied scientifically at least thirty years earlier.

Equally, the idea that prior to the breakthrough everyone saw sleep as a quiescent state of rest is incorrect. When Freud published his *Interpretation of Dreams* in 1899, the whole book was predicated on the idea of an intense psychical activity throughout the night, and that sleep is a state that has to be both engineered and maintained. It was less a question of 'I fall asleep' than of 'I make myself sleep', and Freud devoted hundreds of pages to describing and analysing the psyche's nocturnal activity and reviewing the earlier literature. German sleep researchers had come up with many of the ideas that we see today in the pages of neuroscience journals, yet this history has been more or less forgotten, probably due to a combination of aversion to German scholarship after the war, and the fact that later researchers couldn't read the language.

The assumption that EEG studies of sleep had to await the REM breakthrough is also misleading, and the young doctor Zelda Teplitz had already composed an important and neglected review of EEG studies of sleep and dreams in 1943. Sleep EEG was hardly a new phenomenon, and EEG itself was becoming recognised as increasingly significant. Faith in electrical recordings was initially bolstered by the discovery in the 1930s that epilepsy was associated with a characteristic three-per-second spike and wave pattern, and this would later reinforce the idea that specific functions – or lack thereof – could be linked to the sleep stages demarcated by EEG.

Brain-wave readings were depicted everywhere, not just in scientific journals but in the newspapers, the movies and on TV. States of mind were believed to correlate with EEG data, and in one widely publicised episode, the experimenter predicted from an EEG reading that the subject, a reporter, was checking through his answer to a mathematical problem. Wired up to the apparatus, he was asked to relax until the EEG showed alpha rhythm, and then set his mind to the maths question. He left alpha when he pondered the problem, and then returned to it, before leaving again, at which point the experimenter whispered to his colleagues that the subject must be checking through. The uncritical enthusiasm that such theatre demonstrated is very similar to that displayed today, when results from neuroscience are advertised as giving the mechanisms of cognitive or emotional aspects of our lives.

Although this is largely forgotten today, EEG was once taken to offer diagnoses of personality types or even compatibility of romantic partners, in a way that is almost identical to how brain imagery is so often convoked in the contemporary world. The colourful images of brains 'lighting up' that feature in both scientific journals and the media, however, are hardly ever direct illustrations of what they are supposed to depict, just as brain 'waves' cannot seriously be deemed to depict specific thoughts or character traits. The multicoloured brains are not pictures but statistical maps, and the brain that we 'see' is not the actual brain of the subject of the experiment but an image generated using a statistical template. This sort of functional mapping of the brain is often assumed to be a snapshot, in the way that an X-ray would be, whereas these technologies are, up until today, quite different.

Unlike a camera, functional brain scanning is not a real-time or an optical technology, but uses assumptions about the brain in software in order to construct its images. This is not to deny the value of scanning techniques, but to recognise that the image that is presented as a factual representation of some individual brain process is in fact a representation of a set of statistical values. We might be impressed by the bright colours in the scan images, as if they embody discrete processes, yet the use of colour has been highly controversial, as it turns quantitative differences into apparently categorical ones. The patterns of blood oxygenation in the brain that such images track are also only loosely correlated with neuronal activity, and it is a huge and precipitous step to identify them unequivocally with specific mental processes.

The thirst for science to solve the problems of human existence means that scanning techniques have become part of commercial and supposedly scientific ventures to discover truths about human attachment, emotion, religious belief and memory. Since scanning requires a subject who is immobile, restricted and focusing on a simple task, experiments shamelessly reduce complex aspects of human life to brief laboratory-based encounters: watching a cartoon, listening to a list of words, looking at photographs. Certain parts of the brain are deemed 'active' during such tasks, to then reify what are clearly socially constructed categories, be they the 'mental disorder' of the day or the 'emotion' that the researcher needs to pursue to further their career.

The recent denunciations of 'fake news' sadly play into exactly this mindset. The supposedly liberal and enlightened gesture of distinguishing false propaganda and the real hard news has served, indeed, to draw attention away from the fact that, as historians, sociologists and anthropologists have been showing for about 140 years now, the very visibility that is accorded to any news item will depend on social and economic factors. What gets aired and broadcast will depend on a complex set of decisions and choices, and the facts themselves will incorporate meanings and assumptions saturated with cultural values. Some events, one might object, like a death or a volcanic eruption in Hawaii, are just real things, yet *when*, *how*, *how much* and *if* they are reported introduce precisely these values.

It was perhaps no surprise to see that, in the wake of the 'fake news' media storm, many people with little interest in how facts actually come about took to the streets to try to convince the public to renew their faith in science as an antidote to fake news. Rather than encouraging people to explore what is socially constructed within science and to question their faith in experts – which is, after all, what Galileo, Newton and Marie Curie did – it just posits another belief system, which in this instance involved many doctrines that derived from the most reactionary forms of nineteenth-century reductionism. Believe the coloured pictures of brains rather than inform yourselves about how such images are built and what assumptions are included within them!

Sleep and Memory

The 'news' of the discovery of REM in the early 1950s was certainly billed as exactly that, with the popular press and the media promoting the results of the Chicago research. Yet although it was credited to Kleitman and Aserinsky, the work did not just come out of nowhere. Aserinsky in fact would later claim that Kleitman wasn't very interested in it, just supervising from a distance, yet whatever the details of this priority dispute, it was Soviet and not American research that already in the 1920s had focused on the periodic cycles of human sleep.

Although Kleitman – who could read Russian – gives an abbreviated citation of one of these sources, it is never quoted from or properly acknowledged, perhaps a consequence not just of the egos of those involved but of the Cold War, during which much of this work was taking place. The Russian research clearly discerns periodic cycles during sleep in which breathing and heart rate become irregular and eye movement rapid, accompanied by the other motor phenomena that Kleitman and Aserinsky would investigate. So already several decades previously there was a recognition and an interest in periodicities within sleep.

What is so fascinating about these questions of history is that one of the most influential and powerful explanations of sleep itself is that its function is to facilitate and improve human memory. The idea that sleep involves a certain consolidation of memories was well known by the end of the nineteenth century, and memory was taken to be a rich and complex phenomenon. Sleep was seen as a way of ordering and integrating new impressions and ideas received during the day, moving from short- to long-term memory. Yet rather than distinguishing, say, between recollection, reminiscence and memory, as philosophers and psychologists had, by the twenty-first century memory had become increasingly equated with word retrieval. Subjects are presented with lists of words or tasks, they go to sleep, and are then tested on awakening. Variants involve obstructing REM or NREM sleep, fractioning the amount of sleep, and so on, and there have been many different and ingenious experimental designs here.

Despite distinctions between declarative and non-declarative memory, what remains constant is the idea that human memory is reducible to – or at least modelled by – retrieval of words and behavioural sequences, or, as some researchers put it, 'packets of information'. For many sleep researchers, this is of capital importance as evolution relies on us being able to learn new facts that may be important for our survival. Fact consolidation in sleep thus serves an evolutionary purpose. Of course, you can't put human life under a brain scanner, but you can make someone try to learn a list of words. In a well-known experiment, an electrical current is 'seen' to pass back and forth between the hippocampus, identified as a short-term memory storage space, and the larger storage site of the cortex. We are told unequivocally that this 'was shifting fact-based memories from the temporary storage depot (the hippocampus) to a long-term secure vault (the cortex)'. Free space had now been cleared in the hippocampus, and 'Participants awoke with a refreshed capacity to absorb new information within the hippocampus, having relocated yesterday's imprinted experience to a more permanent safe hold.' This was great news, as it meant that 'the learning of new facts could begin again'!

Apart from the wildly unscientific recasting of hypotheses as facts, it is difficult not to see here yet another phantasy, where life is about keeping things clean and emptying out messy and overfilled containers. The brain process is actually identified with 'cleansing' and 'neurological sanitation', and 'the ease of finding important documents on a neatly organised clutter-free desk'. Although there is little evidence that the hippocampus experiences storage problems or that it needs to empty itself out, it is claimed that the subjects were 'fetching' memories from the short-term storage site before they slept, whereas after sleep the 'memories had moved', as 'the same information' was now being retrieved from the neocortex, where the memories were now living safely. Sleep, we are told, was 'future-proofing' those memories. As this happens day in day out, the hippocampus is cleared out and made ready for the new imprinting of facts.

When psychologists and neuroscientists study behaviour, it is curious how often their conceptions of human life tend to make of it either an exam or a maze. Learning bits of information and then being tested, perhaps with a judgement at its horizon, or observing how rats navigate through a labyrinth are taken as paradigms of almost all purposeful human behaviour, often with a gloss about reward-seeking circuitry in the brain. The idea that human life could be anything other than an exam or a maze seems unthinkable, and we might guess that on this model the goal of human evolution is winning a pub quiz.

It is worth remembering here that exams were for centuries not about recall but the art of disputation, and that the fascination of the maze lay in the point of death at its centre. As the historian of memory Jocelyn Small points out, one of the most pervasive myths about human learning systems is that they involved verbatim recall. On the contrary, she shows, they were most often about thematic recollection, with very little emphasis put on precise formal recall, a fact that much of the early-twentieth-century research into memory also demonstrated. A poet would not be expected to recite an earlier work word for word, but rather theme for theme. And yet this phantasy – that life, or memory, is about collecting new facts – has a dominant place in sleep and memory research, muting any real approach to the richness of the phenomena being studied.

We might contrast this with our own experience, in which much of human life, on the contrary, shows how people do not learn anything, but simply repeat the same painful mistakes time and time again. Should we tell them that there is something wrong with their brain, or that they are not sleeping properly and so failing to consolidate new facts? Women have often observed here how certain men will indeed spend their lives searching for new facts, yet at the same time forgetting about anything that could be called a relationship. It is a pity to see

69

such an exciting field as sleep research become enslaved to the impoverished phantasies of a few male researchers, yet the public thirst for 'science' is so powerful that it may well succeed in obstructing other traditions and perspectives.

———

By the early 1960s, researchers were already warning of the collapse of proper research into studies of retention and recall, a reductionism that essentially redefined what memory was taken to be: a retrieval and storage system for little packets of information, for storing facts that we need for our survival. We could contrast this with the whole of world literature. From the Brontës to Proust, from Homer to Dickinson, a memory is not like an object that can be lost and found, but something that can saturate and texture every aspect of experience. The classical and Renaissance theories of memory studied by Small and by Frances Yates make memory a kind of architectural space that we live inside, whereas the more recent cognitive theories make of it something that is, on the contrary, inside us.

Such distinctions are made more complex by the fact that memory bridges what might seem to be both internal and external space. From the sixteenth century onwards, wills start to link material objects with previous owners, as if a chest or a bedspread was now the chest or bedspread that had once belonged to a grandparent or parent. Such associations apparently fulfilled no legal purpose, yet testify to an investment in objects as bearers of one's past or history. One of the most dehumanising aspects of prison or hospitalisation in many countries is the removal of one's personal possessions, as if this were to deprive the person of part of their very selfhood that is located in objects.

Science-fiction narratives often include scenes of memory transfer, as if the essentials of a human life could be abstracted and transplanted into another body or receptacle. In the recent *Westworld* remake, endless lives are reduced to a finite set of algorithms contained in books in a vast library. But there is always an excess, something that cannot be included, a remainder that is not absorbed in a set of declarative sentences but is inscribed and embodied in objects. Memory here is less about storage or the retrieval of a fact than about how we use and invest things, a process that is operating constantly and not confined to conspicuous moments like the Proustian madeleine or some keepsake that acts as a conduit to bittersweet aspects of one's past. Technology obviously expands this network, as phones and computers form a part of a continuous effort to localise difficult and sometimes overwhelming experiences into images and words.

Memory systems of the classical and Renaissance periods often traced their inception to the story of Simonides, the Greek poet who was attending a dinner when the ceiling collapsed. Nearly all of the guests were killed, and it was difficult to infer their identities from the mangled remains. Simonides, however, could attach names to the crushed bodies because he remembered where each of them had been positioned before the accident. Thus their spatial location was used as a memory device 'for those who would train this part of their mind', and the association between spatial position and words would become the principle of the construction of later mnemonic systems: 'the order of the places would preserve the order of the things'. At the horizon of word retrieval here is a traumatic loss of life and a series of crumpled bodies.

This link of memory to trauma and loss can hardly be studied with word-retrieval experiments, and we could contrast their reductive model with the complexity of a real person's memory. Cultural changes in how memory is conceived exert a subtle pressure here on our actual experience, where we might expect that a memory needs to be like a still photograph, or a Super 8 film, or a frightening flashback, or a selfie. People are often unsure, indeed, if they are 'really' remembering something or whether they are thinking of a photograph they have seen or an anecdote they have heard about their childhood.

As they elaborate their thoughts in analysis, recollections, dreams and sometimes new symptoms come to inflect this, and a sense of history can be slowly constructed. What we see so often in clinical work is how a memory can seem either like an abstract piece of imagery, void of any affective charge, or felt with an unbearable intensity. But in both cases, the person may come to inhabit the memory in a new way, which means effectively coming to situate themselves within it differently. The memory of an assault in childhood, for example, may always have been experienced with a single emotional interpretation, as if the person were guilty of an action that was their own fault, due, perhaps, to a badness within. Inhabiting the memory may involve a reinterpretation: it was the other that was at fault and not themselves.

In some cases, such repositionings involve more than just a re-ascription of blame and even a different identification of the figures present or of the chronology within their life. A scene that they experienced as a participant may turn out to become one in which they were a witness, or a childhood phobia may be resituated after a separation from a loved one rather than before. These rewritings are basic to psychoanalysis and many talking therapies, and we see how, after this long and difficult process of inhabiting a memory, it can take on the emotional charge that it lacked until then, or, on the contrary, its intensity may fade.

—

Processes such as this are troubling not only for the person going through them but for a culture in which good and evil, victim and aggressor must be neatly segregated. All good liberals were up in arms about Trump's projected wall with Mexico, as if this concretised racist partitions between the 'good folks' on one side of the wall and the 'bad folks' on the other. Yet the same childish divisions were surely projected onto the man himself, as he became the embodiment of pure evil. When he made his infamous comments about the clashes in Charlottesville, suggesting that in fact there were bad folks in the good folks and good folks in the bad folks, this proved even worse, as it questioned the rigidity of the divisions that perhaps both Trump and some of his detractors require.

Ruth Leys has documented the progressive erasure of the complexity of memory here in its relation with traumatic experience, echoing these categorical divisions between good and bad, inside and outside. Trauma came to be thought of during the later part of the twentieth century as a purely external event affecting an autonomous subject, a shift that is echoed in the movement from guilt to shame. The subject's unconscious involvement in the trauma is excised, as we see in the eclipse of once popular notions like 'identification with the aggressor' and 'survivor guilt'.

Although the first of these concepts was developed before the Second World War, the experience of the concentration camps provided startling verification. Inmates would mimic the verbal and physical aggressions of the SS, and even their 'goals and values'. Hopes for solidarity with what Primo Levi called 'one's companions in misfortune' were also usually dashed: 'there were instead a thousand sealed off monads, and between them a desperate covert and continuous struggle'. The many bestselling camp testimonies of the late 1940s and 50s are now no longer read by the general public, and we perhaps want to know less and less about human behaviour in the camps.

In its place there emerged what we could call a kind of late-capitalist reading of the Holocaust. People survived not because of chance and luck – emphasised by nearly all the early testimonies – but due to resilience and survival skills, concepts that come not from listening to survivors but from the world of business, where they are deemed the qualities one needs to prosper in a competitive marketplace. Where once the testimonies described brutalities and betrayals among inmates, a new emphasis on solidarity and small acts of kindness and generosity began to emerge.

Instead of seeing this as a result of careful study, it indexes a shift in the basic framework of thinking about human subjectivity, which is now recast in terms of the neoliberal marketplace. As Leys observes, rather than deepening the exploration of our unconscious positioning in traumatic events, the new psychologies establish and reinforce a strict dichotomy between victim and agent. This has some quite radical consequences. Phenomena linked to trauma like nightmares and flashbacks are taken to be direct material replicas of what happened, and thus, as Leys notes, 'stand outside all interpretation'. There is no place here for the unconscious, for phantasy or for the compulsion to repeat.

Such evasions are central to the sleep research that we have been discussing. If someone lies awake unable to shake off the return of certain images, or if they are woken by intense and frightening sensations, these may be understood as photograph-like impressions of an event that happened to them. No further interpretation is required, as if there is nothing further to explain or understand. And once these night-time phenomena are taken to be direct imprints of experience, what could be more logical than to favour their removal?

A sleep hygienist like Matthew Walker advocates quite unequivocally memory deletion, telling us that his hope is 'to develop accurate methods for selectively weakening or erasing certain memories from an individual's memory library when there is a confirmed clinical need'. This sort of behavioural hygiene is of course the stuff of innumerable Orwellian fictions, and taps into the segregative logic that underpins some of the most questionable human excesses. It is probably not an accident that the idea of deleting people's memories has been so ubiquitous in the darkest visions of the future, and it begs the question, of course, of who confirms the 'clinical need': the patient, the doctor or the state.

What matters here is not deleting memories, which are mistakenly seen as bits of information, but refinding one's place within memories, which means rewriting them and resituating them within a history. The effort to remove memories has of course been a feature of repressive regimes for many years, from the early Roman attempt to erase all traces of Domitian, to the redrafting of Soviet school books to delete key episodes in history. We could think here of Macbeth's famous words:

> Canst thou not minister to a mind diseased,
> Pluck from the memory a rooted sorrow,
> Raze out the written troubles of the brain,
> And with some sweet oblivious antidote
> Cleanse the stuff'd bosom of that perilous stuff
> Which weighs upon the heart.

This becomes all the more ill-starred when we realise that memories are not like photos stored on a phone but are constantly in the process of being rewritten, as psychologists have shown since the early twentieth century. Unlike some copy of experience, they are reshaped and recrafted, revised and rerouted according to the changing concerns of a life, and what we wish could or should have happened.

It is also problematic to see memory as uniquely the concern of the individual, as it is linked to the social and political spaces that we inhabit. What value will our remembering a tragic loss or disaster have if everyone else in our community or group refuses to acknowledge it? What memory is here will depend on what it is for the Other. As the anthropologists Leslie Dwyer and Degung Santikarma point out, memory cannot be reduced to often facile ideas of remembering and forgetting, as if one were to take a stance against some external event. Interviewing a Balinese man who had lost his brother to the anti-communist cleansing of the 1960s and had himself been imprisoned, they apologised at one point for asking questions that might have upset him. 'It's not you who has made me remember,' he replied. 'I will have these memories until I also am dead. It is these memories that make me know I'm still alive.'

Rather than trying to remove memories, it is a question of giving them a voice, and of allowing these 'written troubles' to be articulated and clarified. There is also another perhaps even more dangerous side to this thinking about memory. NREM sleep, some sleep scientists argue, has the task of 'weeding out and removing unnecessary neural connections', whereas REM sleep operates to 'strengthen' them. Starting with a mass of autobiographical memory, NREM removes superfluous matter, and then REM works to enhance the connections that remain. This is repeated again and again throughout the sleep cycle, which alternates between the 'culling hand' and the work of 'enhancing'. Only the important elements remain, which must be 'strengthened' and enhanced. Now, it is curious to see in this vision the vocabulary of selection, of a kind of naive social Darwinism applied to memory systems, where the weak and superfluous are removed and the important and strong survive. But can't we also hear in this one of the underlying principles of eugenics, which divides elements of human life into the weak and the strong, the superfluous and the necessary?

Such divisions are central to many modern conceptions of sleep and of sleep hygiene. Culling and enhancement were – and still are – of course basic concepts of some of the most regrettable episodes in human history, and so it is disappointing to see sleep hygienists segregate the human species into those who are 'normal' and those who are 'abnormal', even stating with no irony that teenagers do not have 'rational' brains whereas adults do. The sleep-deprived pose a danger to society, whereas sleep allows a 'deep cleansing' of the brain. There are those normal people who thanks to a refreshing sleep can read the world around them rationally, and the abnormal ones who can't. They will be 'inaccurate in their social and emotional comprehension of the world', which is a danger to society as it will lead to 'inappropriate decisions and actions that may have grave consequences'. Well, what could be more reasonable than to get rid of the abnormal ones – by curing them, of course.

Trauma

Finding a traumatic memory is often taken to be like finding the missing piece of a jigsaw puzzle, and both published accounts of clinical cases and media representations of traumatised people enshrine this perspective. Endless thrillers and TV series revolve around a buried trauma that, when it is finally brought to light, explains everything. Although there are undeniably elements from the past that when remembered can allow a radically new understanding of a life, the link between the traumatic memory and a story must often be questioned, and indeed, the very link between trauma and memory.

In many cases, all that remains of a trauma is a detail of the surroundings: the grain of a piece of furniture, the pattern of a wallpaper, the view through a window. What took place there cannot be registered, and all that marks what happened is a contingent detail of the scene that may return in dreams and nightmares for decades. Aristotle advised remembering sequentially, so by remembering the flanking items you can access what is in between, but in these cases it is only the flanking items that can be remembered. This is a bit like the experience of trying to find an important passage in a book. All you can remember is that it was on the top left of the page, but the page number or chapter remain elusive.

Once again, this basic concept is misconstrued by some of today's sleep researchers, despite being recognised by those working in the 1950s and 60s. It is assumed that one's childhood memories will be of emotional events like 'being separated from one's mother or being hit by a car in the street'. Experimenters hoped to show that REM sleep worked to dissociate the emotions from the memory, so that we could keep the 'information' and not be 'crippled' by the emotional force of the events. Subjects are put in an MRI machine and presented with images that the experimenters deemed 'emotional', and cerebral blood oxygenation estimated.

This kind of experiment, which is not uncommon, misses both the fact that people have individual histories – so that what is traumatic for one may not be for another – and the fact of flanking, whereby the trivial or contingent details come to stand in for or cover over the more intense memories. In reality, when I listen to people's accounts of their childhood, the most frequent earliest memories tend to be those with hardly any emotional charge, seemingly random scenes or exchanges that, months or years later, show their connection to more significant material.

In one of the early experiments in 1965, Herman Witkin and Helen Lewis were studying the effect of pre-sleep stimuli on dreaming, and showed their male subjects different films: a graphic record of childbirth, in which a vacuum extractor is inserted into a woman's vagina and the blood-soaked gloved hands of an obstetrician seen pulling on a chain protruding from it, followed by an episiotomy; a horrific documentary about circumcision, in which an incision is made on the ventral surface of the penis with a sharp stone, and the bleeding member then held over a fire; a film of a mother monkey eating her dead baby as she drags the body around by its legs; and a pleasant travelogue describing the social and economic characteristics of the American Far West.

Their first subject, after watching the childbirth film, dreamt of college kids in a park, with a group of girls wearing white clothes and long white gloves. Bees were pollinating flowers, and the girls didn't want the boys to see their arms and elbows. After the third film, one of the subjects had a clear image of a frog in a pool of water, as if 'it were actually before me'. This had a resonance for him, as he remembered being cruel to frogs as a child, throwing them across a brick-wall incinerator and killing them. Another subject, after the monkey film, dreamt that his mother was telling him about having friends round for dinner and he noted with perplexity that he and his mother were the same age. Both the cannibalistic motif and the age difference in the film had thus been inverted, just as the pure white gloves covered over their blood-soaked palimpsest.

Witkin and Lewis found many symbolic references to impregnation and delivery after the graphic films, and concluded that the recall of dreams was more difficult when the pre-sleep elements were so disturbing. Symbolisation processes had a density here that made the dreams seem more opaque and resistant to meaning than those that followed the travelogue, as if more encryption had to take place. They also argued, with other researchers, that a lack of dream reports is indicative less of a failure to dream than of a failure to recall, and they noted how several of their subjects were unable to recognise dreams that they had themselves reported not long before.

These experiments sometimes tell us more about the experimenters than they do about their subject matter. Where Lewis and Witkin were sensitive to the fact that how an image or a word will affect someone can never be known or predicted in advance, today the reverse is often the case. To posit images that are intrinsically disturbing or happy is to assume that all humans are alike. Yet a violent scene can terrify one person and leave another untouched, or even aroused. What matters here is that person's history, and the positions they have taken in the differing situations that they have been involved in.

After the fall of President Suharto's dictatorship in 1998, advocacy groups in Bali tried to organise some form of group therapy for victims of the anti-communist purges of the mid 1960s, which had seen the murder of between 5 and 8 per cent of the population, and the assault and imprisonment of tens of thousands of others. All that was available was the services of an American franchise, selling stress-reduction techniques to the local population. But when instructed to achieve inner peace through visualising a white sandy beach, many people found this imagery disturbing: they were, after all, fishermen, and what the sea meant to them was radically different from what it might mean to someone in an American city.

How we react to trauma – and what trauma might be – will differ from one person to the next, just as it has been redefined historically. During the American Civil War, irritable heart was seen as the key symptom of war trauma, whereas in the First World War it was shell shock. In the Second World War it was combat fatigue, and with Vietnam came post-traumatic stress disorder (PTSD), which required symptoms linked to reliving the trauma, an avoidance of stimuli associated with it, numbing of responsiveness, and hyperarousal, which could be seen in sleep problems and excessive vigilance. However helpful such diagnoses might be for some, others may be unable to access help because their symptoms don't fit. According to one estimate, around 75 per cent of people who have been through trauma in wartime do not have PTSD symptoms yet still continue to suffer.

Just as how we conceive of sleep shapes how we define sleep disorders, so how we think of trauma will affect how we define categories like PTSD. Whereas historically the medical emphasis has been on physical symptoms, today it is increasingly on memory and its apparent disturbances. The old idea that REM sleep facilitates the transfer of daytime experience and memories held in short-term storage to long-term memory has been used here to explain some of the phenomena associated with this category. PTSD, it is argued, is what happens when trauma remains stuck in short-term memory, allowing rapid triggering and recall through environmental cues. When you hear the doorbell or any sudden and unanticipated noise, it returns you instantly to the battlefield.

The traumatic memories need to go to the other storage system, and sleep, we are told, is what can make this happen. But the evidence here is complicated by the fact that what is supposedly trapped in short-term memory – experienced in the form of flashbacks and perhaps nightmares – is often something that has not actually happened to the person. The sensation of being trapped under rubble from an explosion, for example, might return in the flashbacks, but they were never actually trapped under rubble. What is depicted as absolutely real has not necessarily been experienced. And curiously, when Vietnam veterans describe their abduction by aliens, they show more of the physiological responses we would associate with trauma – such as increased heart rate, perspiration and rapid breathing – than when they are speaking of their experiences during combat.

The question of trauma is complex here. We often find that, indeed, the most invasive memories are actually those that the person has heard about from a friend, an acquaintance or even a TV programme. Faced with an unbearable and unthinkable experience, it is someone else's memory that is put into that place. It acts as a marker for something even more horrifying, and the person can wake up in absolute terror for years with this borrowed memory. One of my patients described a scene in which, as a young girl, she had been touched sexually by her stepfather. The details were precise, the context and location crystal clear. But after some time in analysis, she realised that the scene was actually imported almost wholesale from a close friend, who had described her own abuse by her stepfather after her parents had separated. This ready-made scene had gone into the place of a trauma that she had lived herself but that was much less available, marked only by a handful of sensory fragments.

A well-known example of such a borrowed memory is Ronald Reagan's reminiscence of a wartime episode that he described during his election campaign in 1980.

He told the story of how a bomber had been evacuated after it had been hit, and how the young gunner at the back of the plane was too seriously wounded to bail out with the rest of the crew. Reagan welled up with tears as he quoted the pilot's words: 'Never mind. We'll ride it down together.' It turned out that the story was taken from a 1944 film, *A Wing and a Prayer*, yet the memory had become Reagan's own.

Just as a borrowed memory can take the place of something unthinkable and unbearable, so can certain images, especially those that seem possessed of an absolute beauty. Joseph Robertson, who fought with the US 30th Infantry in the Battle of the Bulge, describes how he had been hiding behind a fallen tree, and could see German soldiers in the field in front of him. One of them, a young boy, was crawling along a ditch directly towards him, and when he was a mere three feet away, Robertson screamed at him to surrender. The boy raised his gun, but Robertson shot first. That night he slept, but for the rest of his long life he was haunted by the image of the blue-eyed, fair-skinned blonde soldier he had killed, 'so handsome, like a little angel'. More than fifty years later, he would still wake up every night crying at what he called the 'saddest moment of my life', marked by this image of utter and devastating beauty.

The image here – like the borrowed memory – is a place-holder, indexing a point of inconceivable horror. Sometimes, trying to access this point can itself be dangerous and unhelpful for the person and there are many cases where it is wiser to mark the place of a trauma than to try to force it into some form of ready memory or narrative. Circumscribing a trauma is different from trying to remember one, and many literary and artistic compositions show us how a work of inscription, of making a mark, is different from a work of representing.

There are very real stakes to these theories of trauma and memory. Asylum-seekers in many countries have to present a coherent narrative of their experience in order to gain refugee status, a requirement that conflicts with some of the basic aspects of trauma that we have discussed. It is an irony that the police forces of these very same countries often recognise that when the account of an alleged victim of rape or assault is always identical, its veracity may be questioned. Trauma involves a fracturing of subjectivity, a rupturing of physical and psychical boundaries that will not produce a nice neat story, but rather, one with contradictions, inconsistencies and errors. And in the place of unrepresentable pain, we can at times borrow the memories and experiences of others.

———

This question of trauma can also tell us something about sleep. Clinicians know that when traumatic events start to become inscribed in dreams, this is a moment of progress, signalling that some form of psychical change is taking place. A patient was aware that when he was three years old, his parents had separated, and that it had been a year until he next saw his father. His mother had packed him and his siblings into the car and off they had gone, with no prior warning or preparation. There were no memories of this collapse of the family, and it was reconstructed from what an elder sibling had explained to him some years later. He could remember the gift that he had received from his father when they were reunited, but nothing more. At a particular moment in his analysis, he began a cycle of dreams that revolved around approaching an empty house, which he now recognised as his childhood home. The feelings of emptiness and desolation were unbearable, yet they were linked now to his history, rather than emerging out of the blue in his daily life in the form of incapacitating depressions.

It is interesting to note how clinical experience runs counter to some of the academic research here, where it is claimed that low dream recall correlates with better social functioning in, say, Vietnam veterans or Holocaust survivors. This begs the question, of course, of how we understand adaptation to society, usually measured in functional terms (do they have a job, are they married, etc.), or in the degree to which the person complains or not about their situation. When we read that Holocaust survivors who don't remember their dreams have 'better long-term adaptation' than those who do, one may also wonder how well their children have adapted. What is blocked out or uninscribed for one generation tends to return with a renewed ferocity for the next, or, as physicians noted after the war, in the form of often chronic somatic symptoms.

So what function does the dream have here? A psychoanalytic answer echoes in many ways the ideas of the earlier sleep researchers, who saw dreaming as an operation on memories. But this is a very particular kind of operation, which takes the residues of the day and binds them to unconscious trains of thought and phantasies. Sleep is a form of 'individual psychotherapy', as one of Freud's students put it, where the unconscious is a reader, interpreting new material and absorbing it in pre-existing structures. That is why it is very difficult for most people to learn anything from experience, and why we tend to spend our lives stuck in the same old ways, repeating the same patterns or mistakes, regardless of whether this is a source of misery or of satisfaction.

To illustrate this, think of the refugee crisis in 2015. The thousands of deaths at sea when flimsy and overcrowded boats from North Africa and Syria sank didn't seem to bother people that much until the appearance of a front-page image of a figure on a beach in Turkey carrying a lifeless child in his arms. The sudden transformation of the alien and unpalatable refugees into the Christian image of the pietà rendered it now a human catastrophe, and suddenly people cared. It was as if the Christian myth had framed the trauma and given it a new status. What was both rejected and often scorned and despised became familiar, and could stir up conventional reactions of outrage.

We could also evoke the dream of the white gloves that we mentioned earlier. The dreamer had watched a film that was probably upsetting, replete with injury detail and graphic depictions of the genitals of the opposite sex. But the dream, in inverting the blood-soaked gloves of the obstetrician into the beautiful white gloves of the girls in the park, was not just denying or sanitising. The dreamer remembered afterwards that he had once offered to buy his wife red gloves to match a dress for a wedding, which she had rejected. The black gloves that he subsequently bought her were lost, and the friends who had got married were felt to be more successful than he was. Themes of loss, reparation and failure thus underwrote the treatment of the 'new' material of the film.

And this is perhaps what the unconscious does during our sleep, inscribing what is disturbing and new into the structures that have been formed during our childhood. And when it can't do this, we may encounter some of the phenomena associated with PTSD, although we should remember here that people who have experienced a trauma are not obliged to conform to what the modern diagnosis requires. If dreaming binds daytime experiences to unconscious complexes, it is interpreting and reading. What can't be read then traumatises, sometimes emerging with terrifying clarity in NREM sleep in the form of night terrors and other violent phenomena.

This would also explain the fact that whereas hardly anyone enters sleep with REM, apart from infants, narcoleptics and those taking certain drugs, traumatised veterans quite frequently display this unusual torsion of the sleep cycle. REM can occur soon after sleep begins or at sleep onset itself, suggesting to some researchers that there is a pressure to dream: in other words, to try to process what has torn them apart. It may also provide a clue as to why night terrors usually fade during later childhood: as unconscious phantasies become established, they can absorb experiences and information that may before then have seemed enigmatic and uninterpretable, like filters that shape new material to their own form.

Dreaming

We cannot avoid the question here of the link between dreaming and REM sleep. When we evoke the swiftly occurring REM of the traumatised veteran, for example, are we being too hasty in equating this immediately with dreaming as such? Rapid eye movement and dreams have been associated for centuries, and it had been suggested long before Aserinsky and Kleitman's work that the movements might correspond to the scanning of dream images. Just as we move our eyes when awake to look at the world around us, so we supposedly move our eyes in dreams as we follow their narrative. Graduate student William Dement joined Kleitman's team to conduct experiments on this and other questions related to dreaming, and the initial results seemed exciting.

Once eye movements were scrutinised so carefully, their direction and speed were taken to indicate a scanning process. If they moved from side to side during REM sleep and then the wakened subject explained that they had been dreaming about a ping-pong match, this seemed proof of the link between eye movement and the hallucinated imagery. Body motility was also invoked, and Dement reports watching his wife's legs moving vigorously in REM sleep and, upon awakening, her description of a dream in which she was performing a lively dance. In another widely cited example, the subject's eyes were moving upwards sequentially and they then detailed a dream about ascending a flight of stairs.

After some years, however, most people gave up this belief in a correlation between eye movements and dream visualisation. Matching reports were often difficult to come by, despite the lucky strike of the ping-pong and stairway dreams, and the fact that newborns, premature babies and those born blind had extensive REM periods seemed to refute or weaken the hypothesis that they were scanning a visual experience. The violent and consistent twisting of eyeballs in some cases is also difficult to reconcile with any viewing experience that we might have in waking life.

Likewise, groups of puppies reared in darkness and exposed to light–dark cycles all showed similar REM activity, suggesting an endogenous programme. It seemed more likely to some researchers that these rapid movements were either effects of random neural firing or the result of some other process, perhaps a kind of neurological work-up to prepare the infant for future learning. The intense REM activity of newborns, indeed, is often taken to be an activation process for the nascent nervous system, promoting growth and plasticity of the brain before more varied sensory experiences become available.

Another massive problem with the scanning idea had been obvious though unnoticed from the start. To take the ping-pong or stairway examples, eye movements during REM are correlated with the back-and-forth or ascending scanning movements of eyes in the waking state. If there is no match, then the eye movements don't fit the dream. But the fallacy here is that if you actually look at what someone's eyes are doing during a ping-pong match or when they are walking up stairs when awake, they don't move from side to side or up and down. They only really do that in cartoons, and in waking life we are moving our eyes in many different directions during such activities.

Dement, once so excited at the scanning hypothesis, would abandon it some years later, although the process of questioning it did produce some interesting results. Susan Weiner and Howard Ehrlichman observed that eye movements become far more rapid when someone is trying to interpret the meaning of a proverb than when they are scanning a visual figure. Another team would find that if rapid eye movement did not correlate with following dream images, its speed would increase notably when the person was not scanning an image but, on the contrary, trying to suppress one. REM, in this sense, could be linked to the effort to make sense of something or to not see something, rather than with some sort of simple sensory tracking. Indeed, in everyday life, it is well known that if you are overcome with anxiety, you might try to focus visually on an external object in order to get through your experience.

A patient described how an acute feeling of unease and then panic started to overwhelm him during a night out in the West End. He left his friends, with no idea of what to do or which direction to go in until he passed a cinema, and the title of one of the films – *Never Let Me Go* – seemed significant to him. He went in and during the film tried intently to scrutinise every area of the screen, as if 'I was inspecting a painting at the National Gallery'. It was only this continuous and painstaking scanning activity that could allay the anxiety. The eye movements here are an index less of what he was looking at than, on the contrary, of what he was avoiding. We might wonder here if this kind of process is indeed one of the reasons why people binge-watch TV: we focus visually on a screen to keep anxiety at bay.

—

If the scanning hypothesis proved doubtful, what other link was there between REM and dreaming? The obvious connection was dream recall. Dement and Kleitman's early experiment found that 79 per cent of awakenings from REM sleep were followed by dream recall, compared to a mere 7 per cent from NREM, and very soon another study found 85 per cent and 0 per cent recall respectively. This seemed like a neat result, which reinforced the separation of REM and NREM sleep. The problem was that it wasn't quite so neat. NREM awakenings did produce dream reports, which many researchers played down as 'mentation' rather than dreaming, arguing that the material was clearer, shorter, more conceptual, less visual, more everyday, less story-like and more plausible.

But this was also put in question. Work at other sleep labs found that there were plenty of NREM dream reports that did not conform to these criteria. As for the frequency of recall, experiments where a fake report by a noted sleep investigator was circulated stating that a drug was found to increase NREM recall did in fact produce this effect. Dream recall was also found to be affected by the sex of the experimenter, and subjects could even be induced to increase dream recall by financial incentives. Reading through paper after paper, we see researchers either desperate to keep REM and NREM separate or to recognise commonalities, a fact that perhaps reflects the personal proclivities of those involved.

Not so long ago, a new theory of NREM dreaming put it down to 'covert REM' activity, operating below the radar against a background of 'atypical physiology', which essentially meant brain activity that couldn't be snugly fitted into tidy sleep-stage divisions. Some of the evidence for this was linked with transitional periods where traditional sleep-stage scoring techniques – which are based on separations – were untenable. But rather than questioning the basic paradigm of scoring and separating, it was in itself a 'covert' way of maintaining the REM–NREM binary, with REM identified with dreaming sleep. In the same vein, dream recall following NREM has even been explained as the memory of dreams from preceding REM states – but never the other way round.

Other variables were also relevant here. One study claimed that gentle waking produced more 'thought-like' material, whereas abrupt awakening generated more 'dream-like' material. But perhaps what was happening here was less the discovery of a real difference than a redefining of what was meant by dreaming. Some years ago I organised a conference on dreams, bringing together clinicians and artists. At the start of the panel discussion, a neuroscientist made some remarks that brought out this shift very clearly. He singled out some familiar Dalí paintings as dream-like, excluding the entire series of other images that had been presented that day, which in fact had been inspired by night-time dreaming. In this sanitisation, a dream was something that was odd, bizarre, illogical, filled with bright colours and impossible happenings. Some dreams, of course, may seem like this, but there are plenty that don't, and the equation of dreams exclusively with surrealist-type fantasies is unhelpful.

———

Even the idea that a dream must be visual is open to question. I was struck many years ago when first reading *Jane Eyre* by Charlotte Brontë's description of her character lying awake anxiously at night: 'A dream had scarcely approached my ear, when it fled affrighted, scared by a marrow-freezing incident enough.' Although the book contains other references to the visual quality of Jane's dreams, here it is unambiguously aural. Indeed, early sleep researchers were interested in the muscle activity of the middle ear, especially during REM sleep, as this seemed to be operating as if it were listening in the waking state. This was present in close to 85 per cent of REM and also just prior to it. Contractions of these ear muscles were even proposed as a more reliable indicator of REM sleep than the eye movements themselves.

Although Kleitman and Dement initially saw rapid eye movements as the criterion of dreaming, they later argued that it was not eye movement but solely EEG tracings. If certain generalisations can be made about the differences between NREM and REM recall, there are always counter-examples, and nearly all studies fail by not giving enough value to the variability of individual dreamers. Even hard and fast rules about the sequencing of REM and NREM are not always instantiated, with

Kleitman himself failing to experience an REM period in the place where his data on sleep stages predicted it with certainty. Rather than simply seeing NREM dreaming as the poor cousin of REM, we might hypothesise that what goes on here is part of a process that will extend to REM. As several studies indeed showed, material from NREM and REM awakenings on the same night often show a similar motif, treated from different angles and in different ways.

In one experiment, subjects were hypnotised and asked to describe their dream while it was taking place. Most of them managed to do this, and on comparing the accounts given during sleep and those elicited after they awoke, they tended to match up pretty well. If this indicated that the dreams that were remembered were indeed the dreams that had been narrated during sleep, the surprise was that there were no rapid eye movements at any time during the descriptions. The dreams, it seemed, had come from another place.

In his well-known work on sleep and dreams, David Foulkes aimed initially to find where REM dreams actually started. But as he pushed awakenings further and further back from REM, he found that there was no point at which dream recall ceased. Abandoning the idea that there would be a moment in REM when dreaming began, he came to see it as a process that continued throughout sleep. Later research would find that even Stage 4 NREM, once believed to be the deepest and most recall-resistant phase of NREM, would produce plenty of dreams that were not very different from those associated with REM.

This continuity implies that a 'dreamwork' is taking

place – perhaps a process of reading, as we suggested earlier – that extends throughout the night and in which disturbing and unanticipated elements may be linked to unconscious themes and motifs. What we imagine to be a localised dream may just be some part of this much more extended sequence. This brings us back to the question of the relation between REM and NREM sleep. NREM almost always precedes REM in the sleep cycle, and its timing seems to be regulated by the amount of prior NREM. But should we then see REM as a kind of treatment or elaboration of what is being processed in NREM, an attempt to save NREM, or a temporary failure to sustain NREM? In other words, is REM a breakdown of some other state or process, a repair mechanism, or a logical development of this in its own right?

These questions could be inverted if we choose to see things developmentally, where it has been claimed that REM is more 'primitive' than NREM, which only really emerges later in the newborn's life. NREM could then be an attempt to treat those disturbing elements that ultimately surface in REM sleep. We can only be in NREM for a limited amount of time – one or two hours – which suggests that it may be difficult for us to sustain. Sleep is certainly a cyclical process, with four or five periods of emergence from NREM to a stage similar to our initial 'drowsiness'. Things need to become more active with REM usually for at least ten minutes before the quiet can be re-established, yet the transition here to REM is frequently interrupted.

Although NREM sleep is so often called 'quiet' here, it is possible that its deep, slow waves have been completely misunderstood. Several researchers have found 'GSR storms' during NREM, periods of sustained and intense arousal signalled by electrodermal activity. Likewise, the horrific night terrors of childhood and occasionally of adulthood emerge only from Stage 4 NREM, perhaps making the highly symbolised dream products associated with REM seem tame by comparison. The longer and deeper the slow-wave NREM sleep here, the more intense the night terror. This may also suggest that processes of symbolisation – that is, encryption and disguise – are denser in REM, and that hence, despite the rapid eye movements, breathing and cardiac accelerations, it is in fact the 'quieter' sleep.

The psychical activity of NREM sleep is much more difficult to remember than that of REM, which is one of the reasons why many researchers chose to believe that there was just less of it. If people who speak during NREM are woken up, they tend to have no memory of what they have said or even that they were speaking, yet if woken from REM sleep they may well remember dreams and fragments of speech. This may suggest, once again, that NREM sleep has more to hide, operating with intensities that, if rendered conscious, may be difficult to bear.

The relation of the signs of physiological arousal with what we might conjecture is happening psychically is very complex here, and there are no neat answers. If someone is tossing and turning frantically in their sleep and awakens to describe a nightmare, it would seem obvious to equate the fast, irregular breathing, accelerated heart rate and sweating with their dream. But there are well-documented examples where the most dreadful nightmare occurs during what appears to be a physiological calm. A doctor fell asleep while lying on a ballistocardiograph table, and after a few minutes woke from a nightmare in which his brakes failed while parking. The car was careering down a driveway towards his house as he tried desperately to reach for the emergency brake. He described his unbearable anxiety and palpitations, yet the measurements of blood pressure, heart rate and the ballistocardiogram showed no changes whatsoever. The only thing to be recorded was a little twitch in his left hand.

We tend to equate the experience of anxiety with bodily changes such as sweating and an increase in heart rate, yet here it seems to be dissociated from its physiology. The involvement of the body and its musculature are indeed closely linked to the REM–NREM question. Oddly, the early work of Kleitman, Aserinsky and Dement always emphasised bodily motility in REM and its absence in NREM. 'In every case', the first two authors wrote, 'the eye motility periods were associated with peaks of overt body activity.' Yet later definitions of REM sleep state that, apart from the involuntary muscles used in necessary functions such as breathing, the body is more or less paralysed. It is true that muscle tone drops strikingly in REM sleep, and certain reflex responses are abolished, yet in the 1930s increase in arm muscle voltage was taken as a sign of dreaming, and there are more small body movements in REM than elsewhere in sleep. Larger movements can also occur, and were once taken to signify scene changes in a dream. The general idea was that the wider loss of muscle tone prevented the acting-out of dreams, as if the dream itself required the inhibition of movement as its condition.

It is interesting to observe here that in narcolepsy, a condition involving acute daytime sleepiness, there can be a similar abrupt loss of muscle tone, called cataplexy, and that this often occurs at emotional moments: entering an argument, initiating sex, raising one's arm to strike a child. The body may slump and fall dramatically although the person remains awake: 'like a puppet with all the strings gone', as one sufferer put it. It would not be rocket science to infer that the inhibition blocks the highly charged action, and if it is true that people with narcolepsy frequently enter sleep with REM, as has been claimed, this would perhaps suggest that REM does indeed involve some kind of shutting-down of the musculature that would allow a disturbing or unacceptable impulse to be played out.

Any approach to these questions would also need to explain why the first and briefest REM period of the night is often 'missed', and if it does occur can be interspersed with brief periods of NREM with spindles or transitory waking before the next phase maybe an hour and a half later. It has even been argued here that since each REM phase during a night's sleep is physiologically dissimilar, it may serve different functions. The fact that many of the phenomena associated with REM, such as irregular pulse and respiration, and genital erection or engorgement, actually begin just prior to it perhaps indicate that NREM is breaking up and cannot be perpetuated without the treatment provided by REM. The claim that poor sleepers spend less time in REM might echo this, together with the idea that the narcoleptic superimposition of REM onto waking states at moments of intense emotion acts as a kind of treatment or attempt at processing.

A sleep researcher in analysis described how he had woken up from a dream with the sudden realisation that he had understood the difference between REM and NREM sleep. He was confronting the head of his sleep lab in a darkened room. There was an accusation that he had taken some documents, and he felt threatened. Running out, he fled through the building until he came to a safe space, and found himself surrounded by people who shared similar views to him. On the other side of the space was a dangerous zone where the confederates of his boss hovered menacingly. He had the sense that three spaces were clearly demarcated. When I asked him which space was the REM and which the NREM, his immediate answer was that the safe, intermediate space was the REM and the dark, dangerous spaces were the NREM, but by his next session, he had changed his mind . . .

Freud on Dreams

Freud believed that the factors that disturb our sleep are exactly the same as those that lie behind our dreams. If we can understand something about the causes of dreams, then what interrupts or obstructs our sleep may become clearer. Freud's theory of dreams is almost always misunderstood or caricatured, yet the basic premise is very simple. Thinking operates at many levels, and as well as our conscious deliberations there are preconscious and unconscious processes continually at work within us. Preconscious thoughts are those that are able to become conscious, whereas unconscious trains of thought usually cannot. Some of these will be formed by an exclusion from consciousness, motivated in part by their incompatibility with other thoughts. They will gravitate around motifs of sexuality and violence, and we can only infer their presence from dreams, symptoms, slips of the tongue, blunders and glitches.

Now, Freud recognised like everyone else that dreams so often seem to revolve around issues and problems we faced during the preceding day. But he argued that appearances are deceptive here. When we dream, an unconscious train of thought will latch onto the preconscious one, smuggling itself in like a stowaway or a hitchhiker grabbing a ride. The preconscious thoughts here may be about things we haven't done properly or are about to do and are worried about: an exam, a visit to the dentist, some work intrigue, our care for a loved one, emails we haven't replied to.

We might then dream that we are sitting the exam or visiting the dentist, and to hasty readers of Freud – or most often those who have never bothered to read him – this illustrates the theory that a dream is the fulfilment of a wish. We do well in the exam, the dental work is painless, and so on. The fact that so many dreams, on the contrary, represent a failure in the exam or a bloody tooth extraction is then taken to mean that Freud's theory is refuted, yet this is exactly what he is not claiming. Any variant of the preconscious thought can be elaborated by the dream, but the key is the unconscious thought that hides with it, which will be disguised to elude psychical censorship.

Freud thought that one of the conditions of sleep is a lowering of internal censorship, which then creates the danger situation whereby unconscious elements risk emerging. A 'dreamwork' will take place, involving encryption mechanisms such as condensation, in which several ideas converge on one image or word; displacement, in which there is a shift of emphasis from one element to another; and secondary revision, which introduces a false coherence or glossing to breaks and fractures. If disguise is so central to dream construction, the key elements will often be the most discreet: the colour of the dentist's chair, the quality of the light, the grain of the exam desk. It is these details that will lead, by association, to the unconscious material that has been smuggled into the dream.

There is thus a difference between the dream wish and the dream desire. The wish may become conscious, and have links to everyday problems and difficulties, whereas the desire must be inferred from the dreamer's associations. These will be absolutely individual, formed in the unique history of each person, a fact ignored by nearly all the experiments that have tried to assess Freudian dream theory. In one of the most exemplary misconstruals, Ancel Keys studied the effects of prolonged starvation during the Second World War, to find no special increase in dreams about food and drink among his volunteers. Later experiments would follow this model, depriving their subjects of fluid in the hope of finding an increase in dreams about quenching a thirst.

The mistake here is to confuse the conscious or preconscious wish (for fluids) and the unconscious desire (whatever it might be, depending on the individual). Freud perhaps encouraged this misprision with his famous anchovy-induced dream, which he included in *The Interpretation of Dreams*. Whenever he eats anchovies or highly salted food in the evenings, he says, he will be woken up in the night after a dream in which he is taking great gulps of water. 'The thirst', says Freud, 'gives rise to a wish to drink, and the dream shows me that wish fulfilled.' This widely quoted extract actually occurs in a chapter before Freud sets out his dream theory, which overturns his own explanation of the dream.

The more comprehensive theory would see the fulfilment of the wish to drink water as an alibi, to draw attention away from unconscious desire, indexed in the dream by a detail of the vessel from which he drank, or some other trivial feature. But this desire is elusive. It is not equivalent to a declarative sentence like 'I want to drink water' or 'I want to murder my siblings'. The desire that analysis is after can rarely be reduced to a single meaningful sentence, but resides in the gaps in between sentences. This is because, in most instances, it could never be fully assumed or articulated by the person in question. They were never really able to have the thought.

Even the simplest dream may conceal this dimension. Dement reports entering his daughter's room when she was under two years old and noted the rapid eye movement in her sleep. Suddenly she said, 'Pick me! Pick me!' He woke her and she immediately exclaimed, 'Oh Daddy, I was a flower.' The key here isn't so much the fact that a flower is something that can be picked, but that there is an ambiguity in 'Pick me!' that may signify simultaneously 'Choose me!' The unconscious thematic of being chosen over her sibling or over one of her parents by the other was perhaps disguised in the innocuous flower dream.

Mythology and fairy tales are filled with examples of this process. In the story of Theseus and the Minotaur, the hero promises his father that he will change the sail of his ship if he is successful in his mission. But after killing the beast, he forgets his pledge, and his father, seeing the ship's old sail on the horizon, throws himself off a cliff. So we have two relations: 'A son deliberately kills a non-human who isn't kin' and 'A son accidentally kills a human who is kin'. Freudian desire is equivalent not to one or the other of these sentences but to the relation between them, where we could conjecture the deliberate wish to kill human kin.

To take another example, in the story of Little Red

Riding Hood, her mother tells her not to talk to strangers on the route to visit her grandmother. She disobeys by talking to the wolf, but then avoids speaking to the woodcutter who will eventually save her. Once again we have a series of relations: 'A daughter disobeys a prohibition by talking to a dangerous non-human' and 'A daughter obeys a prohibition by not talking to a safe human'. In between we could guess that there lies a dangerous desire between a girl and an older man.

Desire here can never be fully assimilated to a meaningful declarative proposition, but resides rather in the contradictions and inconsistencies between them. A dream is like a treatment of a problem, creating different configurations and permutations of material around an impossible point. This could involve desire and also traces of traumatic experience – or both. In many cases, it can come to offer an interpretation of a relationship, bringing out how we relate to some significant Other and how they relate to us.

In a remarkable note to *The Interpretation of Dreams*, Freud observes that 'a dreamer in relation to his dream wishes can only be compared to an amalgamation of two separate people who are linked by some important common element'. What might bring satisfaction to one brings anxiety to the other. Dreams, indeed, are often a response to what is unconsciously perceived as the desire of some Other – almost always parental – be it to absorb, fetishise, feed, swallow, annihilate, undermine, enjoy or abandon us. A dream can articulate and clarify this desire – in which case it may well be frightening and anxiety-provoking – or signal a shift in our relation to it, which means that we may feel relief or a certain detachment.

During a period of great suffering, as she waited for a certain man to contact her who remained silent, a woman dreamt that her father was throwing a ball down from a balcony. 'It could hurt anyone down below,' she said, 'but he didn't care.' In her associations, she remembered a scene several years previously in which a massage therapist told her that her neck pain was caused by the thought that someone was hurting her. To relieve the pain, the therapist advised imagining it as a ball floating away. In the dream, as she realised, her father was the one who could hurt people and, indeed, who didn't care. If the ball needed to float up, he was throwing it back down.

The dream was thus both an aperture onto her sense of how her father related to her and a commentary on her current situation. The man she waited for was just prolonging her suffering, following the paternal template. Unlike many dreams, this one did not require any interpretation as it was itself an interpretation, as the dreamer understood. It was showing her the structure of her predicament, and, interestingly, a series of dreams that followed played out different possibilities of changing her position. In one, she waited in pain after others left her, and in another she set out to find them and was able to ask them about their absence.

How far we are here from the story of the anchovies or, indeed, from the many facile reductions of Freud's thinking. To take a recent example, Matthew Walker's debunking of Freudian psychoanalysis is as follows: he asks someone in his class to share a dream; he listens to the dream, then 'looks intensely and knowingly' at the student, nodding his head, and says, 'I know exactly what your dream is about.' After a long pause, he delivers an interpretation: 'Your dream is about time, and more specifically about not having enough time to do the things you really want to do in life.' The student and the class seem convinced, and he then tells them that he always makes the same interpretation whatever the dream. This is taken to be a scientific refutation of Freudian dream theory.

What is really at stake here? The showmanship simply allows a professor to affirm his superiority to his students, where he is the one who knows and they are not. Even revealing the stock nature of the interpretation just aims to reinforce his position of knowledge over the dumb students, and in this sense all the experiment shows is how suggestion and power can operate in human groups. This is the very opposite of analysis, where the patient is helped to realise that they are the one who knows and the analyst from the outset abdicates from any position of knowledge or expertise. That is why there are no 'experts' in psychoanalysis, only a motley collection of misfits who hope not to impress their patients with knowledge but, on the contrary, to learn from them.

—

After *The Interpretation of Dreams* was published in 1899, all of Freud's subsequent contributions tended to treat the question not of dream interpretation but of the handling of dreams. He was anxious to temper the zeal for dream interpretation evinced in some of his students, and to collapse what he called 'the exaggerated respect' that had been accorded them. Although dreams were certainly the vehicle of hidden meanings, analysts had to give up their passion for discovering some blinding revelation if their work was to be conducted properly. A dream, he said, could never be fully interpreted, and just as there were no set rules for reading dreams, there was no lexicon of dream symbols. All would depend on each individual dream within the context of each individual person's analysis.

There is an important difference here between the meaning and the function of dreams. On this latter question, Freud believed at first that the purpose of the dream is to conserve sleep. It does this by acting on both the external and internal factors that would otherwise keep us awake: problematic aspects of everyday life will form part of the dream, and unconscious trains of thought will connect with them, albeit in hidden and disguised form. Since what is repressed 'does not obey the wish to sleep', a complex operation has to occur to stop us from remaining awake. Freud argued that because the internal factors are threatening and pose a risk to us, they undergo the censorship that works to form the dream. This is the process of disguise and encryption that constructs the dream.

A man in analysis woke up from his sleep to remember simply the single pristine image of a lemon. Although he had no immediate associations to this strange apparition, and was puzzled by it, several weeks later a recollection came to him: when he was five, he had been present when the son of a domestic in his family home had declared that his girlfriend's vagina had become unduly stretched due to all the sex they were having, and that he had tried to make it contract by squirting lemon juice inside it, despite her protests. The motifs of scopic, sadistic or masochistic pleasure – whatever they might have been – had been both reduced to and replaced by the spartan dream image.

We should remember that by censorship Freud does not mean a little fellow who sits in your head and decides what can and can't be allowed into consciousness. It is rather a structural process, like a compression, that results from what can and can't be thought. What is curious here is how difficult it is not to add a thinker, and hence the idea that someone – a thinker – must judge what can be thought and what can't. But psychical censorship is very different. In the example above, we might guess that the boy didn't have the thought 'I am enjoying watching this act of sexual aggression' or 'A woman is being punished for her sexual enjoyment', but that, where the thought could not be formed, the image of the lemon was constructed instead.

It is during the process of falling asleep that this question is perhaps most acute for us. As we let our thoughts wander, they may take disturbing directions, before being encrypted by the dreamwork. Woken up suddenly by his partner, a man was horrified to admit that the split-second image of touching his mother's naked body had been in his mind, followed almost instantaneously by that of a baked dish of sweet potatoes and mussels. The one had seemed absolutely proximate to the other, yet he could make no sense of any connection until, describing the strange confection, he said, 'It's two things that shouldn't be together', an elegant and precise encapsulation of the Oedipal wish.

The dreamwork had presumably transformed the

dangerous and sensual thought into the image of the cooked dish, and it is significant that he could initially make no sense of this at all, a sign that censorship was working effectively. If the meaning were transparent, the ciphering process would have failed. Associating to the image, sweet potatoes and mussels both proved to have links to childhood memories and to the male and female body, but these would only emerge after a careful analytic work. Note also how the thought itself did not wake him up, and we might wonder how it is possible for such sequences to take place.

I think that this is the most obscure and least studied area of sleep, since it is just so difficult to grasp the connection between the parts of the mental process here. If we are woken up, we might remember an image or a thought, but the passage from one element to the next is almost impossible to grasp. Introspection is limited, and the speed of forgetting is astonishing. And yet this is the moment when we are effectively falling asleep, so presumably the opacity of the connection must be a part of the process itself.

To take another example, a woman was woken up by the seat-belt announcement on a plane, and was able, with great effort, to remember the psychical sequence that had taken place in the split second she had dozed off. It recapitulated a thought she had had earlier that day, of how beyond the many reproaches she had to her mother for showing her naked body lay a comparable accusation of her father, followed by the image of the plan of a city. The city was seen from above, with an area distinguished by lines radiating outward, which 'I knew was my father', and then, a bit further away, a 'sort of statue or pillar, which I knew was my mother'. The image was viewed as if a camera were panning out, with the maternal statue very small and isolated in comparison with the 'much larger paternal area'.

What is so striking about the sequence is how a thought is transformed into a visual image, which, we might guess, if she had not been woken, would have been totally forgotten, or absorbed in a dream. Without any knowledge of the connection between the prior thought and the image, it would perhaps have been resistant to interpretation, just another meaningless visual fragment. This can certainly illustrate censorship, as the initial thought was clearly troubling and had only emerged during an analytic session that day. The visual image was a metamorphosis of the thought, disguising it beyond recognition. If the risk of allowing such thoughts seems excessive, it may be the swiftness of the encryption that saves us.

But sometimes the risk is too great. If the disturbing elements are just too strong or too present, says Freud, we forgo sleep altogether. Instead of distortion and disguise, we choose insomnia: we wake up, abandoning the state of sleep. The anxiety that we feel at these moments is the experience of the proximity of the unconscious – or what cannot be absorbed within it – and most people are familiar with this waking in the night in a state of panic or dread. Freud adds that for some, insomnia is an almost intentional state, as falling asleep would itself open them up to these risks of the weakening of censorship. So rather than waking, they may fail to fall asleep in the first place.

What stops us from sleeping is thus also what will wake us up: the most disturbing point of the unconscious thoughts. The key here is to avoid confusing the preconscious and the unconscious thoughts, a mistake made by many of the well-intentioned therapies for insomnia. Treating the day-to-day worries and helping the person to relax may have a therapeutic value, but will not fundamentally affect the sleep issues, as the root cause here lies with the unconscious – or what cannot be assimilated to it – which is simply using day-to-day issues to find expression. This doesn't make things any easier, of course, as the unconscious material is difficult to access and to change. Let's take an example discussed by Freud in *The Interpretation of Dreams* to see how these different elements are intertwined.

A father had been watching over his sick child for days and nights. After the child's death, he went into the next room to lie down, leaving the door open so that he could see into the room where the child's body lay surrounded by tall candles. An old man had been hired to watch over the body, and sat there murmuring prayers. It was in this context that the father fell asleep and had the following dream. 'His child was standing beside his bed, caught him by the arm and whispered to him reproachfully: "Father, don't you see I'm burning?"' He woke up to see a glare from the next room: the old man had fallen asleep and the wrappings of one of the child's arms had been burned by a candle that had fallen onto it.

Now at one level, says Freud, the dream is simple enough to explain. The glare of light shone into the sleeping father's eyes and alerted him to the fact that a candle had fallen. And so he awoke to the terrible scene. But the difficulty is that he did not wake up immediately: in between perception (of the glare) and consciousness (of the fire), there was the dream. The external stimulus (the glare) was woven into the dream without waking him up instantly, and it is here that the unconscious part of the dream is situated.

In his commentary on the dream, Lacan suggests that it is not really the glare from the fire that wakes the father up, but rather something unbearable in the father–son relation, a point of reproach, perhaps linked to a guilt the father bore towards the son. Although the question 'Father, don't you see I'm burning?' refers at one level to the fire itself, and beyond that perhaps to the real of death masked by the image of the flame, at another it evokes the son's eternal reproach to the father for having failed him. Although we don't know anything else about the dreamer and his son, it brings out these two different levels to the dream: the manifest and more superficial level that concerns the actual situation of the dreamer, and the hidden, unconscious level that involves feelings and thoughts that the dreamer may never be fully aware of and that may be too intense to bear consciously.

———

So why didn't the dreamer wake up immediately when he sensed the glare from the next room? Freud suggests that it was to allow his dead son to live just a little bit longer in the dream, but that 'other wishes, originating from the repressed, probably escape us', as we don't know anything more about the context. It may be linked to the opportunity afforded by the accident itself. Could this have given him a way of representing his own guilt and pain, taken up in the dream in the terrible moment when the son grasps his arm? The moment of waking, then, will come as a consequence not of the glare but of the acute and unbearable nature of this pain. The sensory stimulus is secondary to the psychical stimulus.

We could think here of the shock ending of Brian De Palma's 1976 movie *Carrie*. After a carnage of murder and revenge for her humiliation at the high-school prom, the student kills her own mother, before burning to death herself in their home. Her classmate Sue, who had played a part in Carrie's bullying, visits the grave to lay flowers. As she bends down to place them, a hand springs out of the ground and grabs her, like the son's unrelenting grip in the burning-child dream. Sue awakens, and we realise that it was all a dream, but a dream that contained something more real than her actual reality: a materialisation of her friend's deadly claim on her and the point of guilt that lay beyond this.

During the First World War, it was not uncommon for shell-shocked soldiers to willingly lie awake in order to avoid the risks of a dream taking them back to some dreadful point of anguish. Where films like *Carrie* use this to create a twist, it becomes the basic principle of the *Nightmare on Elm Street* series, in which the supernatural killer Freddy carries out his homicides within the characters' dreams themselves. Accordingly, he can only be sought and vanquished within those same dreams: the stakes of life and death are thus situated not in waking life but in the realm of sleep and dreams, closer to us than any shared, external reality.

These examples also show how the many philosophical musings about the blurred boundaries between sleeping and waking may not always be just vague metaphors. The psychoanalyst Lawrence Kubie suggested, indeed, that we are never fully awake, just as we are never fully asleep, an observation that many of the biologically oriented sleep researchers of the 1950s and 60s made efforts to demonstrate. For Kubie, the barriers between the sleeping and waking state are relative and not absolute, with 'parts of us asleep when we are awake and parts awake when we are asleep'. After the 'discovery' of REM sleep cycles, several claims were made that the same cycles also occur during our waking hours, and that the EEG patterns do not always afford such hard and fast distinctions between the two states.

Although many of these arguments are far-fetched, the idea that we are always in some kind of waking state is not altogether implausible. Mothers can wake to the tiniest sound of their child stirring, just as a father may wake to the humming of his mobile while sleeping through his child's cries. In the days before bleepers and mobiles, hospital interns would awake to the tannoy sound sequence 1,1234 but not to 1,123 or 1,12345. There is no doubt that if it is sometimes possible to sleep with one's eyes open, we always sleep with our ears open. Where lab experiments would show this, sleep researchers could also actually witness the mathematician Norbert Wiener asleep and snoring on conference panels, only to suddenly open his eyes and make comments that were absolutely pertinent to the discussion.

Differences between waking and sleeping are indeed not always as categorical as we might like them to be. We tend to take for granted what it means to be awake when a rigorous definition is in fact hard to come by. 'Having one's eyes open' is not really a candidate, as this can occur during sleep and other states where conscious-ness is extinguished. In one experiment, the sleeping subject had his eyes pulled open and a 150-watt bulb shone directly into them, while the researcher waved his hand to and fro: there was no EEG change and no sign of awakening.

The idea of 'attention' or 'contact with reality' once seemed plausible, but this was soon admitted to be fanci-ful, as most people, when subjected to tests, turned out not to be in contact with reality. Supposedly relevant or important stimuli were ignored, and thoughts would wander in bizarre directions, mixed freely with phan-tasy material. Listening to a scientific lecture, doctors described their real thought processes and it was diffi-cult to reconcile these with what might be expected from being 'awake'. One imagined shooting a gun at the face of each of the portraits in the room; one imagined that he would die and his soul fly through the keyhole with a loud whistling noise; one imagined suddenly levi-tating and hovering over the table to the shock of all attending; and one imagined that the head and upper torso of a portrait would come to life.

The idea of 'attention', likewise, is hardly synonym-ous with being awake, as selective and directed focus may be precisely what we employ to protect ourselves from pain and anxiety. If we feel overwhelmed or uneasy, we tend to use attention in this sense of paying attention 'to something', whether it is work-related or a recreational activity. There is often a leaflet at the back of aircraft seats that advises directing attention to some object within the cabin to overcome sickness or fear. The focus keeps our mind away from other elements that may be disturbing us, so attention may be equated less with wakefulness than with defence, perhaps defence against the same disturbing elements that sleep must contend with.

Equally, the idea that we are constantly asleep, only woken occasionally by traumatic breaches of our defensive systems, is also attractive. Those engaged in rhythmic and monotonous activities like sustained, slow moving to traditional dance bands can actually show an EEG of light sleep. Soldiers have been known to fall asleep on long marches yet continue their stride, and the sleep researcher Ian Oswald walked around Edinburgh for a considerable time with a volunteer on either side of him, with closed eyes and technically in the state of sleep.

Young people today speak of being 'woke' to issues and problems, as if the standard state is simply being asleep. Lacan indeed thought that the father who had the dream of his burning child only woke so as to continue sleeping. We could contrast this with Viktor Frankl's account of his experience of the concentration camp nightmare. In his once widely read book *Man's Search for Meaning*, he describes how one night at Auschwitz he witnessed another prisoner thrash around repeatedly during his sleep. Frankl moved to wake him with a comforting gesture, but then 'drew back the hand that was ready to shake him'. He knew that this would be a mistake: the horror of the camp to which he would awaken, he believed, would be worse than anything that a human reverie could conjure up. He left him to the nightmares.

Sleep and Language

We have seen how for Freud, just as disturbing elements can wake us up, they can at times be a motive to avoid sleep altogether. Yet this is almost always opposed to our conscious volition. We want to sleep, and the conflict between this wish and our inability to sleep can seem dreadful. Insomniacs know, however, that the actual wish can in itself block sleep. The very focus of the psyche on the wish to sleep evokes a kind of self-hypnosis, and the equation of sleep with a hypnotic state was once popular. Even today sleeping pills are called 'hypnotics' – from the Greek *hypnos*, meaning 'sleep' – and in public shows of hypnotism the subject is so often told, 'Now you are going into a deep sleep . . .'

The paradox here is very simple. Wishing to sleep becomes a focus of our attention, yet to sleep we need to withdraw attention from thoughts and wishes. Thus the more we try to sleep, the less we are able to. As Dickens put it, 'We cannot help thinking that the very anxiety to sleep is one of the principal causes of insomnia.' This circular process is finely described by Lee Scrivner in his history of insomnia, whereby it is the wish to sleep that ultimately obstructs sleep. The many therapies of insomnia that instruct us to think about something – a sandy beach, an empty white room – thus risk keeping us awake, as, despite the monotony and the repetition designed to soothe us, they still require the mind to focus on something. Insomnia's therapy, says Scrivner, is its cause. As the poet John Suckling said of sleep, 'The more I court it, the more it flies me.'

In many cases, sleep here comes to embody the object that the person desires, not because of any original valorisation but simply because it becomes what is unattainable. As the person longs for sleep week after week, month after month, everything now seems to revolve around it, and visits to doctors or therapists all crystallise sleep as one's ultimate aspiration. The person anticipates during the day that he will not be able to sleep at night, worries about the effects of this, and scrutinises himself anxiously as he lies down, just as the next morning he calculates the hours he has lain awake. Insomnia – in the sense not only of the actual staying awake at night but also of the daily discourse around it – becomes a form of desire, and this fact alone can make it even more difficult to shift. Something else has to take its place, which is why love often has beneficial effects in such cases.

The paradoxical fact that the wish to sleep can keep us awake also opens up another apparent paradox. Lying awake at night without being able to turn off our thoughts suggests that in order to sleep, thoughts need to be somehow muted. When we look closer, the thoughts here tend to have verbal form, yet in so many instances it is precisely words that are necessary in order to initiate sleep. Robert Burton, in his *Anatomy of Melancholy*, recommended 'to read some pleasant author till he be asleep', and the American physician Joseph Collins concludes his popular 1912 book, *Sleep and the Sleepless*, with a chapter on 'Reading as a Soporific', pointing out that books are the most common instrument that insomniacs use to 'purge the mind' of the thoughts that trouble them.

Books, he says, are chosen as 'an opiate', and each reader must choose the right book 'to displace vagrant, insistent and harassing thoughts'. 'I have to get myself out of my own mind in order to sleep,' one insomniac says, 'and books are the only way.' Just as children may appeal for a bedtime story, so, as adults, books allow an escape from what would otherwise keep us awake. Yet only a few decades after Collins published his advice, publishers were complaining that as effective sleeping pills became easily available, sales of fiction decreased. What could allow language to be replaced so easily by a drug? And how can words help us to transition into sleep?

The psychoanalyst Vincent Dachy writes of the way that bedtime stories are 'craftily created to raise a level of stress only to appease you just before anxiety would have settled in'. The tension of narrative keeps the much more terrifying threat of sleep – and what it involves – at bay, both distracting us and preparing us for it. And bedtime books can certainly offer treatments of the themes and motifs that may plague us: love, separation and death, to name the most obvious. But is there also something beyond the actual content of such stories that affects us here and helps us to fall asleep?

Can the fact that the written words are those of someone else transport us from our own thoughts into another space? Do we need another person's story to be able to separate from our own? Falling asleep, Freud pointed out, is not just about removing stimuli, but about changing our relation to these stimuli. Drawing the curtains, turning off the lights, disrobing, blocking out noise are of course at one level removals of stimuli, but they are also perhaps symbols of this process, metaphors of a passage to another state and of the work of withdrawal. Sleep itself is perfectly capable of occurring when these stimuli remain present, as everyone knows who has lived near a busy road or fallen asleep with the lights on.

Dreams are adept at incorporating the very things that ought to be waking us up, and so one of the conditions of sleep is not the absence of sensory stimuli but the curtailment of our interest in them. But how can our relation to stimuli be changed? In everyday life, mobiles and screens of all sorts embody an ever-present demand, in the specific sense that they address us. We are continually at the receiving end of messages, questions, communications and imperatives. Whatever form they take, they interpellate us, requiring us to reply and respond. And this is an aspect of all human language.

Linguistics traditionally examined three main functions of language: the referential, the emotive and the conative. The referential was about how words referred to objects and created meanings; the emotive described the speaker's relation to their words and the expressive side to language; and the conative treated the relation to one's addressee, such as ordering or questioning. Strikingly, what these areas of study neglected was the actual experience of being spoken to, which is, after all, our situation right from the start of life. Even *in utero* we are spoken both to and about. Yet if as we arrive into the world we are addressed almost without remission, there is very little space to formulate a reply until we develop a system and rhythm of communication with our caregivers.

We can defend ourselves against many aspects of our early dependency, such as being fed or being coerced to do things, but it is much more difficult to defend against this primary experience of being addressed. We can see it in its rawest forms in the hallucinatory experiences described by some psychotic subjects, when they feel that a voice or a look is singling them out, addressing them directly, even if they are unaware of the content of the message. This can also be a mainspring of torture. Everyone knows about the appalling physical conditions and practices of the concentration camps, yet survivors describe the absolute horror of the almost incessant practices of interpellation imposed by the Nazis: roll calls, name checks, inspections, all revolving around the vocal summoning of the inmate. Even if it was clear that the interpellation would not result in death, it was still 'like a stab in the heart' every time.

And it is perhaps this very precise aspect of language that we find on the borders of sleep. Although teddy bears and bits of cloth have attracted more attention as bedtime soothers, words are equally important here. In a pioneering study in the early 1960s, Ruth Weir put a tape recorder next to her two-and-a-half-year-old son Anthony's bed. The 'crib speech' that she analysed was surprising in many ways: it was full of imperatives, as if he was both talking to someone else and appropriating the commands and instructions that he had himself received during the day. Weir argued that these apparent mono-logues were in fact dialogues, as if Anthony were continually addressing himself and his cuddly toy Bobo, which otherwise had little significance for him.

Anthony was in the process of internalising speech,

finding ways of using the pieces of language that had previously had him as their object. Where he was their unique addressee, he was now able, through crib speech, to construct dialogues: in other words, to pass on the place of being addressed. And isn't this what needs to happen to allow our nightly sleep? When we lie awake, desperate to sleep yet unable to turn off our thoughts, it is perhaps in part this aspect of language that assails us: we can't turn off the function of being addressed, of being interpellated or in some sense summoned.

When Freud said that we sleep because we cannot bear the external world 'uninterruptedly', we can understand this in the sense of uninterrupted interpellation, the fact that there is no 'off' button. Although the content of our thoughts is obviously important here – the altercation we had at work, the task we failed to complete, the health of a loved one, the email we didn't send – it is the grip of the thoughts as such that we cannot break. The mobiles, tablets and laptops that may lie by our bedside only materialise and accentuate this interpellation. And this brings us back to the question of why bedtime stories are so effective.

As the Dutch philosopher Jan Linschoten pointed out, the key to the bedtime story is that we do not have to respond to it. A story doesn't ask anything of us, apart from listen, and it is this that sets it apart from so many other experiences of speech in our daily lives. We are constantly required to reply, to respond, to obey, yet here at last is something different. In contrast to the commands and orders and requests that our caregivers make of us, to be taken up in the emails, texts and instructions that we later receive day in, day out, here is a place where, for once, we do not have to take up a position. It is as if the addressee function is turned off, or at least temporarily suspended.

———

This feature of the bedtime story is echoed in another strange nocturnal phenomenon. If we are woken up suddenly while in the process of falling asleep, we may be left with an exceptionally vivid visual image or a word or sentence. One sleep researcher woke to the Joycean sentence 'Or squawns of medication allow me to ungather' and another to the crisp phrase 'Analytical geometry in three dimensions'. These creations often seem poetic: 'The war stands in red marks' or 'I think like water in sapphire' might seem to make little sense but are semantically quite rich. Grammar appears compressed and disjunctive but is not always followed: 'And find that all with syphilis is immediately' or 'They are exposed to verbally interlection'.

Such experiences have often been described and studied, and one thing that they have in common is that very frequently the person is left with a profound sense of the importance of the image or phrase. However mysterious it might seem, it is felt to carry some weight of signification. The elliptical words or the image interpellate them in an acute sense, like a vector of meaning. These hypnagogic phenomena can seem intensely significant, even if we don't know what their meaning is, like the solution to some puzzle or problem that we can no longer remember.

Once we link these odd experiences to the actual process of falling asleep, we can understand them in a new way. If sleep requires a certain separation from the inter-pellative nature of language, from the way in which words and thoughts seize us, perhaps these hypnagogic phenomena are the last gatepost of this function. They are the transition point between being addressed and not being addressed. It is why, after all, they occasion-ally wake us up, as if we are being called upon, and people often awake here to hearing their own name being called out, which is interpellation at its most basic.

Yet most of the time, as students of hypnagogia have pointed out, when we are woken artificially by someone else, rather than awakening ourselves, the words that we recollect are not addressing anyone in particular. If the dream is an 'adventure', it was said, the hypnagogic image is a 'spectacle', which requires no engagement from the sleeper. Yet isn't this duality internal to hypna-gogic phenomena the crucial clue here? We are either woken with a start by words and images that seem important to us, or we feel uninvolved and distant from them. Once we get beyond the gatepost of interpella-tion, sleep will be easier, as speech no longer summons us. When Freud said that to sleep, it is not the presence of stimuli that has to change but our relation to them, it is in this sense of separating from the interpellative, summoning function of language.

This can help us to explain the process of falling asleep, sleeping and then waking. As we fall asleep, there is a weakening or, more precisely, a treatment of the inter-pellative dimension, as we see with crib speech or the bedtime story. While we are sleeping, we have succeeded in avoiding the interpellative function, and when we wake up it is this function that calls us. Indeed, as people wake up, they often actually address themselves – 'Get up!' – in an imperative interpellation, or speak to themselves in a bossy way, a phenomenon that is much rarer when they are trying to initiate sleep, and interestingly, EEG shows an increased sensitivity to sound as we doze off. The traditional psychoanalytic approaches to the question of sleep always tended to focus on the ego, and how it is supposedly decomposed and then recomposed from sleeping to waking, but once we shift the focus to language, a new perspective opens up.

And this can give us a clue as to certain forms of insomnia, in which we are unable to perform this separation from thoughts. Our attention cannot be loosened, and so the thoughts continue to exert their interpellative force. As Coleridge put it, the moment his head hits the pillow 'my thoughts become their own masters'. This can either stop us from falling asleep or, at times, wake us up. What we are unable to separate from is less the thoughts or images themselves, in a sense, than their interpellative dimension. Sleep requires that we are no longer addressed, that thoughts no longer speak *to* us.

Learning to Sleep

If a focus on sleep can prevent sleep, is there another kind of attention that can in fact facilitate or even encourage it? The sociologist of sleep Simon Williams draws attention to an observation made by the philosopher Maurice Merleau-Ponty that opens up some key questions about insomnia here. 'As the faithful in the Dionysian mysteries invoke the god by miming scenes from his life, I call up the visitation of sleep by imitating the breathing and posture of the sleeper . . . There is a moment when sleep "comes", settling on the imitation of itself which I have been offering to it, and I succeed in becoming what I was trying to be.' We sleep, then, by identifying with a sleeper, as if copying what we imagine them to be doing is what actually allows us to become like them. As a patient put it, describing her bedtime ritual: 'You have to pretend to sleep in order to sleep.'

What a strange phenomenon. We can't drive by adopting the body language of the driver or do any number of everyday human activities by mimicking the external physical actions of others, so are we really coaxed into sleep by a process of imitation? People who complain of insomnia often want to sleep as long as another person, as several sleep researchers have pointed out. Merleau-Ponty has noticed something here: when we prepare for sleep, we act as if we are already sleeping, and crucially, this action involves an implicit identification with a sleeper – in other words, with someone else. I think that the emphasis is less on our identification with ourselves as sleeping than with a third party. To sleep, we need to become like someone else who is sleeping.

Although this might seem surprising, doesn't it echo our very first situation in life? For a baby to fall asleep, proximity to the mother's body and attunement to her breathing rhythms may be crucial. As her heartbeat and breathing slow, so do those of the child. Already *in utero*, respiratory rates accelerate when the mother is active and slow down when she is sleeping. Many people, indeed, try to slow their breathing as adults in order to prepare for sleep, as if synchronising their body rhythms to those of a virtual or real companion. In the 1940s, doctors might put the earpieces of their stethoscopes into the ears of sleepless patients and the receivers on their heart to create this effect. Similarly, disruptions in maternal sleep so often impact directly on those of the child, and this continues right through adulthood.

When we talk about a baby's adaptation to the rhythms of day and night over the first few weeks and months of life and their learning to sleep, aren't we really talking about an adaptation to the mother's adaptation to the rhythms of day and night? The way in which a mother's sleeping pattern changes has a reciprocity with that of her child, as we see in the well-known sleep changes that occur around three months. Seasonal variations in light and temperature seem to have little impact on this moment of 'settling' (sleeping through from roughly midnight to 5 a.m.), and infant sleep becomes more robust now. Infants will certainly wake several times during this period, but will swiftly fall back to sleep, and most parents will be unaware that their child has not slept through uninterruptedly.

In an early study, Kleitman had indeed suggested that sleep was a construction, arguing that the changes between ten and fourteen weeks were 'one of the first learned performances', moving from a 'wakefulness of necessity' to a 'wakefulness of choice'. Wakefulness seems most pronounced now when the parents are having their own meals, as if the infant is curious and engaged with what they are doing. During this time, hours of day sleep decrease while hours of night sleep increase, with a reduction in night feeds taking place concurrently. From now till around six or seven months, the mean hours of night sleep tend to be stable.

So there is a change in the distribution of sleep and a new pattern of feeding in which initially irregular patterns of day and night feeding become more organised to follow the day–night cycle. As Kleitman observed, an 'acculturation process' is at play here, and the initial rest–activity cycle of about an hour is 'modified, distorted, and in part abolished' by the adjustment to the diurnal routine of living. We could note here that Kleitman's mothers were mostly following on-demand schedules, whereas only a few decades previously it was quite common for babies to be left screaming without any night feeds, in the hope of an early socialisation.

Later research would also find that the entrainment of the sleep rhythm to the day–night cycle is fused with the interactions with the caregiver. In a series of careful studies, Theodor Hellbrügge showed how circadian periodicity may be built up out of much shorter cycles, with the earliest zeitgebers being maternal touch and stimulation of the mucous membranes. Light and darkness will be secondary to this, and the speech and looks of adults will also occupy an important place in this sequence of establishing bodily rhythms.

This relational aspect is crucial here, and the mother's own sleep–wake cycle will have effects on her adaptation to the baby's perceived cycle. Although she may be following the on-demand pattern of feeding, a mother will be influenced by her own pattern of daily activity and her own emotional particularity. This will affect how she responds to the child, who will pick up on her capacity to respond, her speed of reaction, her interest in the baby's activities, her absences, and the many other subtleties of parental handling. As Sanford Gifford pointed out, the infant is here highly sensitive to how the mother signifies her own wish to sleep or stay awake, and the evolution of the child's sleep rhythm is thus partially mediated through his relationship with her.

The big question is why this sleep pattern appears to stabilise around the three-month period, and why it is also at this time that deep slow-wave sleep starts to emerge, and sleep onset moves from REM to NREM. It might seem obvious that it would correlate with some development in the relation of the child with its mother, and infant researchers have studied the range and quality of interactions here. Clear differences seemed to emerge between the infants who settled by three months and those who did not. At first, the researchers tried to link the number of feeds with the settling pattern, but this was not illuminating. But when they looked not at the feeds but at what surrounded the feeds, they got results: the time spent playing and interacting with the child around the feed was what distinguished the settling from the non-settling group. The more that mother and child elaborated things together, the more that sleep could be established.

Three months is also the age at which many studies have situated the infant's ability to anticipate and postpone, which echoes the relevance of the interactions around feeding. This means that the infant is not overcome by the immediacy of hunger, but can anticipate, knowing that the feed – and the contact that this involves – will come. The number of night feeds is reduced here, as if the infant is more aware of the fact that the mother will not disappear for ever when she leaves him. Many other researchers coming at this age from different angles have all linked it to forms of anticipation, which implies having symbolised something of the mother's absences and registering the fact that she will come back.

This is never a given, and some children are unable to interpret maternal absences as anything other than a bottomless hole or an act of betrayal. They may fail to respond to the mother on her return, staring into space or rocking themselves mechanically. Later in life, the absence of a partner or friend may be experienced as an act of unspeakable cruelty, prompting absolute withdrawal or sometimes reprisal. An operation has to occur here that symbolises and gives some kind of sense to the mother's comings and goings, which will in turn make other separations more bearable. It is possible that this correlates with three-month settling and the ability to sleep through for several hours, and the individual differences in the age of settling would fit well with variations in this process of symbolisation. If this were the case, it would in turn raise other questions: are there forms of insomnia linked to this process? What would happen to sleep if one were never sure of the mother's return? And if she could abandon us, what must we be for her? What is our value?

———

Although there is considerable variability from one child to another, the structure of sleep certainly changes over the course of the first six months of life. René Spitz thought that true sleep only starts after about three months, and even Aserinsky concurred that sleep is not acquired ready-made at birth. He doubted that infants really have REM prior to three months, as their eye movements differed from those of older children and adults, and sleep and wakefulness would need to be segregated out of the baby's puzzling mixture of quiescence and activity, in which REM-like periods can occur when the eyes are both open and closed, and when the infant is sucking, fussing or crying.

These hybrid states will disappear over the first three or so months, and by this time the infant will typically enter sleep with NREM. Half-sleeping, half-waking states tend to fade, and sleep becomes organised into larger units, coordinated with day–night cycles and with feeding patterns. The link between sleeping and feeding here might seem obvious, yet it is bizarrely absent in much of today's research. A World Health Organization report on sleep can tell us that 'A priming of the circadian sleep–wake cycle seems to be organised by the feeding cycle', but the implications of this are unexplored. Looking through paediatric journals and books of the 1950s and 60s, in contrast, early sleep disturbances are almost synonymous with feeding problems. The infant can't settle because they are not being fed, or fed too much or at the wrong time, or too harshly or too feebly.

It is striking to see how case after case of infant insomnia is in fact a case of oral obstruction. The many reports of sleeping difficulties in the first three months seem almost incomprehensible today given the dissemination of information about the feeding needs of the child, yet they show the close link between sleep and food. Timed feeding schedules and guidance about leaving a child to cry without feeding at night are often followed blindly, and much of the work of paediatricians was to counter the 'good advice' that their patients had received from family doctors, the media and relatives. Once again, sleep might be improved by a scepticism directed at what we are told about sleep.

Spitz would argue that true sleep appears when the infant starts to imagine its appetites satisfied in a hallucinatory way, in a basic form of dreaming. Strange as it may seem, many of the early researchers thought that dreams were in some way oral experiences, a hypothesis that echoed the periodicities of sleep. Seeing a baby sucking and mouthing with its eyes closed might well suggest that it is imagining a feed, and to link this with dreams was the logical step. Whatever we make of this, any theory of why we can and can't sleep needs to account for the often pervasive activity of the mouth and jaw during the night, and there are at least two different perspectives here. In the first, the infant hallucinates oral satisfaction in its sleep, and that is why the mouth is so busy. Some researchers claimed that dreaming can also inhibit the physiology of hunger during sleep, so it almost literally takes the place of a feed.

Aserinsky and Kleitman in an early work had linked REM sleep to the intervals between feeds, and noted that the infant would often wake up to be fed at exactly the point where an REM period would be about to start. They cried for the breast initially every hour or so, and then at intervals that were a multiple of the hourly cycle. Yet the infants were not just sleeping neatly between feeds but would cycle between periods of activity and rest. This cycle, it was claimed, might then persist throughout later life, though rather than sleeping for twenty minutes every hour or so, light, noise and social obligations entrain us to a more or less twenty-four-hour cycle, and the initial sixty minutes becomes more like ninety. Although we might sleep for a consolidated eight hours, the old cycle is still there, visible in the recurrent periods of REM sleep.

Kleitman interpreted these results – and later data – as proof of a basic biological cycle of rest–activity, to which hunger and the demand to be fed were to some extent secondary. The periodicity came first, and then the orality. This sixty- and then later ninety-minute cycle length is often confused with circadian rhythm, but represents a process that supposedly operates throughout the day and night, peaking and then dipping, affecting our alertness and then propensity to drift off. Today, some sleep advisers claim that completing these cycles is more important than the actual number of hours spent asleep, and that we tend to wake up at multiples of the ninety-minute period.

Other physiologists understood the cycle to be symptomatic of hunger contractions, and the psychiatrist Roy Whitman linked the number of dreaming periods – taken to be equivalent to REM sleep – to the number of feeds, so that where the number of night feeds goes down, the number of mean hours of sleep per night goes up. Just as feeding would occur for more or less even times throughout the day and night, so distinct REM periods would form within the architecture of sleep, and Whitman argued that they served to supply the oral satisfaction necessary to return once more to a deeper sleep.

Oral wishes would be fulfilled in the REM periods, and hence the dream worked to protect sleep. The sucking movements and jaw activity during sleep were taken to be confirmations of this idea, as was Dement's widely cited notion that dream deprivation results in an increase in appetite. Researchers also noted how a feeding child would have a lot of eye movement despite a relatively quiescent body, and how older children and adults often explained their refusal to sleep as an anxiety that they might miss out on something. Even if they had no concrete idea what this something was, the sense that sleep would mean a deprivation was crystal clear. The oral model explained this: the sleeper really would miss out on something – their next feed.

In a ridiculous experiment, researchers tried to study this link between dreaming and eating by actually substituting the one for the other. The first subject declared his predilection for banana cream pie, which was dutifully baked by the wife of one of the team. After the first bout of REM started, they woke him and gave him a slice. He ate it with great gusto, commenting, 'What a way to do research!' An hour later, they woke him as he entered the next REM period and gave him another slice, which he once again consumed with relish. After three more awakenings, he reported the dream 'I was having a cup of coffee and a cigarette'. He ate the next slice with less enthusiasm, and produced a fifth dream fragment: 'I was given some spaghetti, but I was scraping it off the plate into a garbage can'. The next portion was received with reluctance, to give the sixth dream: 'Dr Dement, I dreamt I was feeding *you* banana cream pie'. If the researchers hoped to find an oral wish, what they got instead was a revenge.

And this introduces the other model of dreaming and orality. The last of the banana pie dreams is clearly a response to the poor man's conditions, reversing the relation between subject and experimenter. He takes the demand to feed him and sends it back to the feeder. In our earliest interactions, the objects we receive – milk, food, etc. – matter not simply as biological inputs but as signs of love. If they have a nutritional value, they are also symbolic of the caregiver's relation to us, as what they have the power to bestow or withhold. The problem here is that once they become signs, they will never be able to nourish us entirely. Their very presence brings with it the possibility of their absence. As bearers of this symbolic dimension, they introduce a lack into the heart of our nutritive transactions.

The breast and the bottle's milk are always more

signs than merely objects of satisfaction, which is why infants and children so often push them away. Frustration, as Lacan argued, is a refusal of this gift, symbolic of both love and its withdrawal, and hence we fall asleep not because we are satisfied, as Freud believed, but because of the disappointment inherent in the symbolic dimension itself. What we receive, as a sign, is never quite enough, and this lack of satisfaction is indexed in many cultures by the bedtime drink or snack, the little object proffered at the transitional moment between waking and sleeping. The ubiquitous sucking and gnashing and grinding of teeth that we find in REM sleep can now be seen as compensations for the symbolic failure.

This symbolic dimension was noticed also by Hartmann in his study of the sleeping pill. As he pointed out, 'People do not take sleeping pills simply because they have insomnia, but because they ask for sleeping pills and someone supplies them.' Taking a sleeping pill is an interaction, which can signify obtaining permission from a parental figure who says, 'It's all right to go to sleep', in the same way that a pregnancy may follow the moment that the green light is finally received from an adoption agency. It can also function as a transitional object or security blanket, a sign that the doctor or ally is somehow present. 'Someone will give me something to show his love, to show me that I am worth something.' The sleeping pill thus 'becomes a gift, a token of love', just as it can be a way of transferring potency, a form of oral impregnation or, indeed, slow suicide.

It is no secret that we inhabit a culture of easy prescribing practices, but the number of people I meet who in their early twenties and thirties are already dependent on sleeping pills is quite shocking. They may obtain the drugs from the web, or go from one private doctor to another to get the script that they need, yet National Health GPs will also sometimes collude, using antidepressants as sleep medicine. What are obviously transitory disturbances of sleep linked to anxiety are medicated with repeat prescriptions, with no proper review. The painter Francis Bacon took sleeping pills every night for at least forty years, and when I asked one of the doctors who prescribed them why they were necessary, he said that he had never asked. Perhaps it is easier to take insomnias as some kind of fact that requires no more unpacking, to protect ourselves from learning too much.

It is particularly troubling in young people, who may never be able to wean themselves from pills that even the most corruptible sleep hygienists recognise as unhelpful and dangerous. There can be a panic at the idea of having run out of pills, and the certainty that sleep would be impossible without them. The pill, as Hartmann observed, can take the place of a transitional object, a condition of going to sleep, and the demand that it is always there perhaps echoes our wish that our caregivers do not abandon us, that they, like the pill, are ever present – or that we have replaced them with something that always needs to be there but that isn't them. For some, the actual pills are never swallowed, yet sleep cannot even be contemplated without knowing that they are to hand. The thought of being without them is the gateway to anguish, just as the repeat prescription brings a relief: we have been given what we need.

The dynamics of giving and asking, of demanding and prescribing, show clearly how we are in a space that is shaped by relational and social processes. A newborn may receive the breast or bottle when it cries as if this were an automatic reaction, but very soon the symbolic side of these transactions is apparent. A cry, after all, is being interpreted as a demand for food or company or a nappy change, and whatever its original motivation, the question of the *meaning* of the response it receives will transform it. We could compare the infant's cry for its mother with what is known as 'The Ask', the moment when fund-raisers and charity workers risk capsizing a carefully established relationship by finally asking for their donation. This demand is so important and so precarious that there are even workshops and seminars that offer instruction on how to perform it, showing how far removed we are from what we may imagine to be the simple, biologically oriented requests of childhood.

This link between feeding, demanding and sleeping is perhaps nowhere as clear as in the night-time trips to the refrigerator that so many insomniacs and night wakers describe. The appeal to food punctuates the night, and may allow either a settling back into sleep, or an exacerbation of guilt at having eaten too much. Many people, indeed, lie awake in bed going over exactly what they have eaten and drunk that day, or carefully plotting what they will eat and drink the next day. The night-time feeds can complicate this even further, as the person may not be sure where they should be situated: with yesterday's intake or tomorrow's.

We could remember here the case described earlier of the young woman who would create her own special time during the night, waking at 3 a.m. and then going back to sleep at 5 a.m., whose flatmates were never aware of her secret. As she spoke about these liminal spaces, she referred several times to her 'greed' for them, and it is perhaps no accident that later, when she sought help, it was for a bulimia that now took the place of the early wakings. A compulsive feeding and a slice of time during the night were homologous.

This connection is echoed in the odd belief that many people seem to share that sharks don't sleep as they are just constantly eating. It is true that some marine mammals are able to sleep unihemispherically, so that one half of the brain sleeps while the other remains awake – at least according to standard EEG measures – which means that they can swim continuously with one eye closed and one flipper inactive. But this is not the same as eating.

This is one of those images that seems to stick in people's minds, and hence must touch on something in us: perhaps the idea that sleep is simply what happens between meals, and that sleeping means not feeding and therefore some kind of deprivation. It would be no surprise to then see thoughts of deprivation cluster so swiftly and easily around sleep: have I slept enough? Have I had the recommended number of hours? Am I being prevented from sleeping? Why is my sleep being stolen from me?

These are exactly the kind of thoughts that we might imagine an infant to have in relation to the breast or bottle: have I been given enough? Why is my feed being curtailed? Is food being stolen from me? The promotion of a norm – eight hours – will only then serve to exacerbate such fears, playing on the unconscious equation between food – or rather, its absence – and sleep. It may also explain the historical popularity of some of the old medical theories of sleep, which posited a reduced blood supply to a hungry brain, as if the latter were a kind of insatiable cerebral mouth.

The link between sleep and deprivation is equally clear in the idea shared by many people that they won't be able to sleep unless they have an orgasm first. Sleep is often associated negatively with sex here: in the stock image, the man falls asleep while the woman wishes to continue an intimacy through talking. The slumber has been interpreted as a traumatic withdrawal, from both the possibility of intimacy and the shock of detumescence, but sleep and orgasm are bound up usually much earlier in the masturbatory practices of childhood and adolescence. Sleep is only possible, the person believes, if they have managed to come, and if for whatever reason this does not happen, sleep is unavailable, broken or abbreviated, with a powerful sense of not having received something. Insomnia becomes the penalty for frustration.

As with food, the key here is the sense of *conditionality*: something has to happen in order for sleep to be possible. Whether this is oral or genital, it demonstrates the tenacity of our sense of entitlement. We must receive something in order to allow sleep, and this requires an external agency to bestow it. Sleep is thus profoundly relational, bound up with our archaic bond to others.

———

These two theories both link dreaming and REM sleep to orality, yet in quite different ways. The first perspective positions the dream as what goes into the place of an object that isn't there: the mother's breast. We dream instead of feeding, with the prototype of the dream being a hallucinated oral satisfaction. The second theory links the dream not to a real absence but to a transformation, the fact that the breast has become a symbolic object. We dream here not instead of feeding but because of feeding. Due to its symbolic status, feeding is never really feeding but always something more – or less.

Both of these hypotheses are illuminating in their own ways. The frequency of feeds cannot be correlated so neatly with REM periods, but the idea of a connection between them is interesting, especially given how the REM-like state of the first few weeks of life will eventually mutate into the more segregated units that we find later. Ronald Harper and his colleagues at UCLA found, indeed, that REM states were much more likely to follow waking with feeding than waking alone in newborns, and they posited a further link between feeding and the sleep cycle.

This REM period would drop sharply twenty minutes after feeding ended, implying that feeds were entraining the cycle of REM and quiet sleep. 'Such an entrainment of the sleep cycle', they conclude, 'indicates that the mother, in regulating feeding time, may also be indirectly modulating sleep cycling in her infant.' This connection is also there right at the start of the Kleitman and Aserinsky research, suggesting an agenda that would be progressively neglected by their Chicago team. As for the symbolic dimension of exchanges with the mother, this is undeniable, although whether it is a cause of sleep seems far from certain. Is sleep always a way to avoid disappointment?

What both perspectives have in common is the idea that sleep is constructed in the place of a lack or absence – however this is theorised – and that it is structured by the experience of longing. The extraordinary ubiquity of experiments in sleep science that involve some form of 'deprivation' – of REM, of NREM, of food, of water, of light, of darkness, of environmental comforts, etc. – might suggest a reflection of this very fact, as if the contours of sleep are defined implicitly by this idea of something being missing, or indeed, forcibly denied or withheld: to find out the truth about sleep, we have to deprive the sleeper in some way. Yet the oral arguments would imply, on the contrary, that sleep is in itself the result of a deprivation.

Sleep would thus have a more or less defensive function, and indeed, many studies show us children who fall asleep almost immediately after experiencing a traumatic or disturbing encounter. Children whose mothers were abruptly hospitalised fell asleep faster and spent longer in deep sleep than others, just as children who had been painfully circumcised without anaesthetic seemed to fall into deep sleep rapidly, countering the researcher's assumption that the pain would result in more crying and wakefulness. Compared with a control group, these infants had a major increase in NREM sleep. Monica, a fifteen-month-old girl who had to be fed through a tube to her stomach due to an oesophageal atresia, was visited by many psychiatrists and physicians interested in her case, and would fall into a deep sleep whenever she wished to avoid contact.

Many of the popular methods of getting babies to sleep have also been interpreted in this way. Programmes whereby the parent either lets the child cry or gradually extends the time they are left crying at bedtime and during the night have often been found to 'improve' sleep. When they work, everyone is happy. But the deep sleep into which the child falls has been associated by critics as precisely this defensive shutting-down: it is not to fall into the nurturing arms of sleep but to desperately switch off as a response to trauma. Will this then mark their sleep for the rest of their lives? And doesn't it suggest that there are different kinds of sleep?

We find this also with older children and adults. During the Second World War, when air raids were a regular occurrence, if the actual attack did not come swiftly after the sirens, an overpowering sleep was often reported. Bizarre as it may seem, soldiers could also fall into a deep sleep while waiting for an imminent attack; Ian Oswald cites the case of a rear gunner on bombing missions who was unable to stay awake as the most dangerous part of the trip approached. One of my patients would fall asleep on the couch almost systematically when he did not want to think about some aspect of his history that had been touched on, and many clinicians have described similar phenomena.

Ethologists also have qualified sleep as a 'displacement activity', noting how birds such as the avocet and the oystercatcher will fall asleep when they are caught between the propensity to attack and to escape. For Spitz, sleep is indeed the template of all defence, an archaic physiological and psychological withdrawal when we are in situations of pain and anguish. Yet we could ask whether staying awake can have the same function. When we read through the many studies of the effects of mother–child interactions on sleep, it is remarkable how often problems and frictions lead to either sleeping deeply or, on the contrary, an inability or refusal to fall asleep, as if the two states were poles of a psychical equation. Several studies have found that children of mothers who reacted harshly to sleep disruptions or encouraged or exaggerated them would either fall asleep almost immediately or be slow to fall asleep.

What sleep research misses out on here is the relational aspect of human development, that we internalise aspects of our relations to others, and this affects us throughout our lives. Just as falling asleep may be linked to the early relation to the mother, so waking up can also be understood as a relational process. When babies and infants awaken, it is often explained as due to hunger, but just as hunger itself is so swiftly bound up with the process of interaction with the caregiver, so awakening is always an awakening *to*. The child may be searching here for contact and dialogue, detaching waking from the simple need for nutrition. And it is surely no accident that people often report their most profound experiences of loss of identity when they awake in a foreign place, as if it is in that split second after waking that we expect to receive the coordinates of who we are.

Waking Up

Waking up is fused from the very start of life to the question of who and what we wake up to. There is obviously a massive difference between waking up to find mother there and waking up to no one. The low spirits and misery that many people experience when they wake up later in life may not just be the result of the expectation of another day of drudgery at the workplace, but to this feeling of someone not being there. If in our earliest months we might wake to find someone there caring for us, or close by, later we wake to her absence. This point of emptiness is swiftly filled up with thoughts of things we have to do, unpleasant duties and chores that at least give some sort of content – negative as it is – to this void.

In the debate around oral theories of dreaming that we discussed earlier, Spitz and some of his colleagues nuanced the initial emphasis on the child's relation to the breast. They argued that during feeding the child spends most of its time looking or trying to look at the mother's face, and this would be a kind of screen onto which dreams were then projected during sleep. The idea is perhaps fanciful, but becomes more interesting when we link it to the question of what we wake up *to*. Indeed, before going to bed and upon waking, most people examine and scrutinise exactly the same part of their body in the bathroom mirror: the face. Could it be that our own image comes into the place here of the face of the mother that we would seek not only in feeding but also at moments of waking? It is perhaps not a co-incidence to hear people sometimes bemoan the fact, as they prepare for bed, that they look just like their mother.

This question of falling asleep *with* and waking *to* also inflects our arrangements for sleep. Childcare thinkers and historians have all commented on the strange emergence of the practice of isolated or 'private' sleeping. Anna Freud pointed out many years ago that the human infant is one of the only mammals which does not sleep in direct contact with the mother's body. And although sleeping in the same room or bed is and has been the most widespread nocturnal situation for most of the world's population, the last 150 years have seen progressive sanctions against it in the West and, increasingly, elsewhere. Infants must sleep separately and, if economic circumstances allow, have the benefit of their own bedroom. This is supposed to both encourage independence and allow the parents to sleep uninterrupted, yet how odd that the infant here is expected to sleep on its own while the parents are so often unable to sleep without each other.

How this question of separation is handled will no doubt have an impact on sleep. If sleep means being without someone else, presumably some sort of confidence in their return and in their proximity is necessary. We saw earlier how being able to anticipate this may be linked to the famous three-month 'settling', and children will soon have other ways to elaborate and symbolise this question. Infant researchers noted how children who wake a lot during the night tended to be those who could often only fall asleep when being rocked or held. The better sleepers were those who did not need to be held or rocked but thumb-sucked or used transitional objects more than the others. They had replaced bodily contact with something else.

Similarly, caregivers of the waking babies held them more frequently and touched them more often, indicating perhaps less a response to the child's distress than a manifestation of their own anxiety or sexuality. They would also respond more rapidly to daytime crying than the mothers of the better sleepers. Isabel Paret observed that mothers who have had separation problems in their own infancy may wish to hold on to their children for longer, to provide the togetherness that they never experienced themselves, just as mothers with strong negative feelings towards their babies may feel reassured if they wake up in the night, to confirm that they are alive and unharmed.

One of my patients dated her sleep problems from the birth of her first child, who she had kept next to her in bed during his first few months. Her mother had warned her of the dangers of co-sleeping, and she would lie awake continuously, imagining what would happen if she were to drop off and roll over onto her child. Years later, she would still remain awake, anxiously awaiting her son's return home from a night out. These difficulties with sleep were only tempered when she was able to start to elaborate her hatred of her son, made all the more difficult by the intense and pervasive love that she felt for him. She felt that he had stolen her life, and failed to become the good little boy that she had hoped for.

In another case, a mother would wake her baby several times a night, explaining this first as a need for companionship, and then as a way of assuring herself that her daughter was alive. The night-time play covered over a terror that became clearer to her when she linked it to her own history: her mother had lost a child before her, and the spectre of the dead baby lay at the horizon of her fears. Interestingly, despite barely sleeping, she did not complain of these gruelling nights. The prospect of not having them seemed far worse to her.

—

It is curious to see how just as some modern child hygiene advocates putting the infant to sleep on its own, so most sleep science insists on isolating the experimental subject. The person is hooked up to EEG and other devices for measuring eye movement, heart rate, respiratory rate and muscle tone, and encouraged to sleep in a single bed. Mummy isn't there, and the subjects are also invariably too embarrassed to run through the complex bedtime rituals that they might require at home. They don't have sex with a bedfellow or masturbate, and yet this entirely artificial subject is the one we expect to give the real facts about sleep.

Similarly, the question of waking up is hardly ever addressed. There must be a difference between waking up and being woken, yet the anger or frustration that this generates is never factored into the research findings. Any parent who has contact with their children would know that waking them up produces reactions and moods quite at odds with those that might follow from awakening at their own pace. It could even be argued that not being woken is itself a part of the definition of sleep. And there is a significant differential between those who are – at times – permitted to wake and those who are not.

On an official visit to Morocco in October 1980, Queen Elizabeth arrived for a state dinner in full regalia only to find the palace closed and no one there to attend to her. A few days later, at her farewell banquet, the palace was indeed open but once again her host, Hassan II, was absent: no one had dared to wake the sleeping king. What might seem an amusing vignette becomes darker when we realise the potential effects of this deference, and military history is replete with instances where soldiers have not dared wake a commanding officer, with tragic consequences.

In the recent film *Passengers*, this question of awakening is even equated quite directly with murder. Thousands of would-be colonists are in deep sleep on their way to a distant planet, yet due to a technical glitch one of them wakes up ninety years too soon. It is not possible for a single person to send themselves back into hibernation, and he knows he will die before the ship reaches its destination. As he ponders his dreadful and lonely fate, he becomes fascinated with one of the sleeping passengers, played by Jennifer Lawrence, and makes the decision to wake her up. What seems like a romance is thus simultaneously a homicide: the act of waking her is effectively an act of murder, as it means that she will now die too before reaching their destination.

The lethal act of waking in *Passengers* saves the protagonist from isolation, and it is no accident that so many of the peculiarities of both infant and adult sleep evoke links with others. The processes that sleep research has studied in infants – such as changes in motility, crying, facial expression, startles, urinating, excretion and mouthing – are spaces where relating takes place, as most of them either occur within interactions or initiate them. They are never just dumb biological behaviours, and the responsiveness of the parent, through speech, touch, looking and feeding will help to shape the neural, autonomic and hormonal functions of the infant. When babies wake at night, they either fall back to sleep or involve a parent in their moment of waking, and how the latter responds – or fails to – may leave its mark upon their sleep patterns.

A woman described how she was always bad-tempered and grumpy in the mornings, resentful at having to wake up and go to work. At one level, what could be more natural? Don't so many of us detest the obligations of early rising and the tasks that follow? But in fact, this everyday sentiment carried its own particular history, which shaped the bitterness of her experience. Her father had favoured her brothers over her, and his death when she was a child had left her mostly with memories of frustration and exclusion. But she remembered that on one unusual day, he had let her sleep, deciding not to wake her for school. When she eventually woke, her siblings had already left and she felt her father's act as an expression of love.

Although it was never repeated, it was perhaps for this exact reason that it mattered so much to her, a single moment when he had chosen her over the others. On that one morning, the requirements of daily life had been forfeited, and she imagined how he would have seen her asleep and come to his decision. For so many years afterwards, this image of love would govern her experience of waking, as if having to get up and prepare for the day was equivalent to negating the very possibility of being lovable. The ordinary and uneventful process of waking had become like a blow to her sense of self, reminding her unconsciously of everything she had lost. Beyond it lay the complexity and depth of a relationship.

Yet the phantasy of the sleep lab is exactly the opposite: that relationships don't count, or if they do, that they need to be minimised or factored out to reach the true biology of the human body. In sleep, however, as the psychoanalyst Mark Kanzer pointed out, we are never truly alone, or we try not to be. We sleep with some sort of index of others, whether it is the child's demand for his parent, the adult's demand for their partner, or the demand for lights, cuddly toys, drinks, snacks, and so on. It is difficult not to notice the fact that in Dement's popular book *Some Must Watch While Some Must Sleep*, there are constant and oddly intrusive illustrations never of the single sleeper but always of a sleeper being watched over by someone else, as if to acknowledge this repressed dimension of sleep research. And indeed, Dement, Kleitman and Aserinsky all used their own children in their experiments, as if they took the place themselves of the watching parent.

We could remember here that when Kleitman isolated himself in 1938 in Mammoth Cave in Kentucky in probably the most famous sleep experiment in the discipline's history, he took his student Bruce Richardson with him. They hoped to see whether they could adapt to a six-day week made up of twenty-eight-hour days in an environment where there were minimal changes in light, temperature and sound. As the University of Chicago's press release put it, they would be free here from external influences such as sunlight, temperature change and . . . 'the activity of others'. But how could Kleitman be free of others if he had taken someone with him?

And in their 140-foot-deep laboratory, they were in fact waited on by staff of the Mammoth Cave Hotel, who would deliver fried chicken and hickory-smoked country ham every day, together with the newspapers and correspondence. Media representations of the experiment depicted the pair almost like castaways, yet 'the activity of others' was there all along. Their interaction would even have direct effects on the experimental procedure, as Kleitman, unwilling to take naps himself, actually forbade Richardson from sleeping outside of their proscribed nine-hour period. So even in the 'isolation' of Mammoth Cave, the mark of human social order was there: a prohibition.

Publishing their results later, Kleitman had been unable to rewire his bodily rhythm, although Richardson had been more successful. We might wonder what the effects of their interactions were on their physiology, and how this close and enforced proximity between an older and a younger man might have affected their sleep and body temperature. The few studies that attend to such details have always found that human interaction does have effects on sleep data, from the sex of the experimenter, to the expectation to produce dreams, to the quantity and frequency of dream recall in both REM and NREM sleep.

When real and sustained isolation takes place, as we find in cases of solitary confinement or self-imposed cave dwelling, a curious feature emerges if there really is no one else there. When Michel Siffre isolated himself for fifty-eight days in a cave with no timepiece and no deliveries of fried chicken, despite increasing physical and psychical distress he found that time was passing quickly. When the day of his release was announced to him shortly before the end of the two-month period that he had set, he refused to believe it. He was convinced that he had about a month more left in the cave. Similar underestimations of time have been reported by prisoners who again, contrary to expectation, are surprised when their confinement term is declared: time had been passing so swiftly that they had anticipated further days or even weeks.

Imprisoned by the Rákosi regime in Budapest in 1949 on espionage charges, Edith Bone observed that during her seven-year incarceration alone in a basement cell, although 'I had read that time dragged in prison I did not find it so, on the contrary it flew too fast. The guards often looked at me wonderingly when I got the evening meal mixed up with the mid-day one and thought supper was lunch.' And Richard Fecteau, during nineteen years in a Chinese jail, of which nine were spent in solitary confinement, would find that time could be abolished through daydreaming, and that hence it passed rapidly. But is isolation really the key factor here?

After the Courrières mining disaster in France in 1906, in which 1,099 miners were killed in a massive explosion, thirteen survivors remained underground in a confined space for almost three weeks, yet were convinced when rescued that it had been only four or five days. Similarly, three brothers who were trapped together under rubble for eighteen days after the Messina earthquake in 1908 estimated the time elapsed as four or five days at most, a fact that attracted the curiosity of contemporary researchers. Experimental studies that followed would confirm this consistent underestimation of time in conditions of sensory isolation or radical removal from the framework of everyday life.

Yet why doesn't time pass more slowly here, as it does for the insomniac lying awake at night, alone with their thoughts? Wouldn't fear and anxiety tend to dilate rather than constrict time? Or is it less about underestimating the time one has actually spent than overestimating the time that one assumes lies ahead? To argue that the person is just disoriented due to an absence of habitual zeitgebers is unhelpful, as in plenty of examples of solitary confinement the cues of regular mealtimes and the day–night cycle are still present. Is it the feeling of helplessness or, more precisely perhaps, the total dependence on the Other, the rescuer or the jailers? If so, this may evoke our earliest situation of dependence on our caregivers, and suggest once again that our sense of time is constructed through our relation with others, and how we are able – or unable – to wait for them.

Recognising these processes can help us to understand more about both sleep and insomnia. Some people find it impossible to be alone, others less so, and how we articulate and make sense of our link with others must have its effects on sleep. It would be far-fetched to imagine that a child who is awoken during the night to attend to its mother or who wakes and calls for her would not ask the question of what it represented for her, or, as analysts put it, what they are for the Other. This burning question of childhood accompanies us throughout our lives, exacerbated, punctuated or attenuated by our professional, romantic and sexual encounters. Are we an object for the Other? Do they really recognise us? Do they hear us? Are we lovable? Can we be desired? Could they abandon us?

In a review of sleep disturbances in children, a Menninger Clinic study noted that the most common parental attitude to children's sleep problems between the ages of one and three was that it reflected the child's concern that they, particularly the mother, would leave them. 'This child's difficulty in falling asleep is that he needs me always present', as one parent put it. The question of their value for the Other is thus central for both the parent and the child, and it is in the knotting of these two sets of concerns that some of the most robust insomnias are established. Each is wondering about the other's question.

A woman with a history of insomnia that had lasted decades described her anguish at bedtime as a child, fearful of the impending separation from her parents. Yet her night-time cries would almost instantly bring her father to her room, as her anxiety was unbearable to him. He would wait just outside her door 'with pursed ears' for the slightest sound from her, and then rush to her rescue. In a nice slip, where she had intended to say that he couldn't bear her not sleeping, she commented, 'He couldn't bear to let me sleep.' Later in life, she would email her parents every day without fail just before going to bed, as if to undo the separation between them.

The daily urgency of this ritual, her conscious guilt at living away from her parents and her fear of being alone were all accentuated by her father's own difficulty with separation. The more that a parent has managed to overcome such anxieties, the easier it may be for a child to overcome them in turn, and to find ways of treating the question 'What am I for the Other?' This may suggest that sleep is made possible by a process of symbolisation of this very issue: the less the child is caught up in the question of what they are for the Other – and hence whether the Other can leave them or not – the better they will sleep, a phenomenon we see also with adults, who often report deep and satisfying sleep after someone has signified their love to them.

If there is an insomnia linked to our inability to separate from interpellation, from the thoughts that assail us, there is another kind of insomnia where we lie awake absolutely unable to sleep yet with no specific rumination or concern. This is the insomnia of pure anxiety. The person often describes a kind of blankness, as if it is the body rather than the work of the mind that is preventing sleep. As the writer Marie Darrieussecq describes it, in this insomnia there is no 'because of': it is an insomnia with no 'reason', just a 'terrifying lucidity'. The experience of time here is less that of clocks and symbolic metrics than that of the object, with the body as one's obstacle, as if an agitation or sense of urgency is encapsulated there. We lie awake waiting for something to happen, as if only some kind of external intervention could save us. That's why the appeal to food or to sleeping pills may seem the only solution.

Perhaps in this kind of insomnia we are suspended from the question of what we are for the Other in its purest form. But we are not thinking, calculating or second-guessing, just reduced to a state of bodily anguish. Many people lie awake at night rehearsing phantasies where they are a star or a hero, which is a way of assuring themselves of a place: they have won a sporting award, saved someone from a traffic accident or thwarted a terrorist attack. In the subsequent moment of adulation or gratitude, they know what they are for the Other. The phantasies thus protect them from a space in which, precisely, they don't know, and it is perhaps this space that we find in the second form of insomnia.

We have succeeded in turning off interpellation, but we have gone from thoughts to something that feels worse: now, there is nothing calling us. The person might explain that they are not worrying about anything yet still they cannot sleep, and a curious detail recurs again and again here. 'It's like being punished for something,' says one insomniac, 'only I don't know what I did.' The vocabulary of punishment just keeps reappearing in descriptions of this most ravaging insomnia, yet, in the absence of a thought, a worry or concern that would render the insomnia rational, there is a disjunction between the punishment and the crime.

Sleep Debt

This question of guilt is pervasive in the interactions of parent and child around sleeping. When there is a disturbance of sleep, the parent so often feels compelled to do something: they must become involved in some way, and it is very common to feel that the failure of the child to settle is their own fault or responsibility. The child is not sleeping because of something that they, the parent, has done wrong. We could note here how parents also often feel punished by their child's sleeping problems, and they may blame themselves for the insomnia, evoking their own unworthiness as a parent or sometimes even their ambivalence towards the child.

While we tend to think of bedtime rituals, emerging in the second and third year of life, as treatments of anxiety, they may also aim at a guilt for both the adult and the child. All human societies contain rituals that bookend sleep, and these are both cultural and idiosyncratic, ranging from a prayer or incantation, to checking that doors are locked and hobs turned off, to moving one's tongue against the teeth in a particular way. Beyond the standard prescriptions of cleaning and then grooming the body, perhaps the two most common requirements are the presence of an object, like a stuffed toy, and some rhythmic movement, such as stroking or rubbing. These are the necessities that frame sleep, and their most obvious quality is their repetitive nature:

they have to be run through and performed prior to any entry into the state of sleep.

Why does sleep require this strange preparation? And why is it that so many people are unable to sleep if their night-time rituals are blocked or compromised? If today we often associate the times before and after sleeping with physical practices, such as brushing our teeth, disrobing and washing, in the early-modern period these preparations were also spiritual. Specific prayers would mark the times before and after sleep, as well as in the 'watching' period between sleeps. There were prayers for undressing, lying down, waking between the two sleeps and morning waking.

The person had to be made ready for the night, as sleep was a special space in which the soul was purified, and one's relation to God was no longer obscured by the distractions of the day. One of the most common medieval prayers, still widely used today, made the connection unequivocal:

> Now I lay me down to sleep
> I pray the Lord my soul to keep.

Sins had to be repented, and devotional texts and objects could be manipulated and handled in this process. It is quite likely that our contemporary practices of washing and brushing derive from this notion of a spiritual purification, as if the bodily exercises were a metaphorical extension of this other kind of cleansing. Washing may thus not have originated in any concern for hygiene but due to moral concerns. Once completed, sleep would be a reward for Christian behaviour. To sleep, we need a clear conscience.

As Thomas Nashe put it in his 1594 pamphlet *The Terrors of the Night*, this time 'is the devil's black book, wherein he recordeth all our transgressions'. The devil 'surrendres to our memories a true bill of parcels of his detestable impieties. The table of our heart is turned to an index of iniquities, and all our thoughts are nothing but texts to condemn us.' This last clause could be inverted today, so that it is all our texts that become thoughts to condemn us, as we pore over our SMS log to mentally rewrite or revise our exchanges. The constant here is the idea that it is around sleep that we mark and enumerate our sins, the many ways in which we have failed or done something wrong.

When George Herbert wrote, 'Summe up at night, what thou hast done by day; / And in the morning, what thou hast to do', evolutionary theorists may read this as a cognitive encouragement to learn new facts that can be consolidated during sleep, but it is more likely linked to a calculus of sin and penitence. The summing-up acts as a catalogue of one's actions, which can be scrutinised and judged, while the rehearsal of one's obligations in the morning aims to ensure a Christian conduct. Sleep was often construed during this period as a means to allay anger and sorrow, as well as this treatment of impurity, but the two operations are not unconnected.

Historians of affect and emotion have shown how different traditions have been at work here, which could be described as the Augustinian and the Stoic. For the latter, passions must ultimately be removed or negated for rational action to take place. Thinking is progressively demarcated from emotion, and is accorded the priority, a split that is echoed in today's cognitive therapies. The

Augustinian tradition, in contrast, does not aim to delete emotions but to give them a direction, a proper orientation. To imitate Christ was to identify with his Passion, allowing an affect such as love to transmute or redirect anger or hatred.

This is very different from the world of the Stoic, for whom optimal performance is linked to the excision of affects. Thus the ideal Stoic in Cicero's *Tusculan Disputations* greets the news of the death of his child with the words: 'I was already aware that I had begotten a mortal.' This detachment is of course belied by the well-known insomnias that so often follow bereavement, and it is intriguing that once again this failure to sleep is linked less to sadness than to guilt. We could think of the reproach to the father in the burning-child dream we discussed earlier, as well as countless literary and filmic examples.

As Kafka put it, 'Sleep is the most innocent creature and sleepless man the most guilty.' Just as for Coleridge lying awake, 'all seemed guilt, remorse or woe', so it is for the grieving father in Freud or the criminal kings in *Henry IV* or *Macbeth*. What keeps them awake is the lack of a clear conscience, the fact that they have blood on their hands, or believe themselves to. Literature has at times linked rejections and disappointments in love to the arrest of sleep, but the motif of guilt is far more frequent. If a clouded conscience inhibits sleep or wakes us during the night, what does that suggest that sleep is in itself? Phrases like 'the sleep of innocents' or 'sleeping like a baby' reinforce this association of sleep with some kind of purity: to sleep like that means that no wrong-doing has occurred.

Should we understand this as simply a consequence of the Christian conception of sleep as purification? Or as something that goes beyond religious tradition? It would be difficult to ignore the fact here that a large percentage of the population can only go to sleep once they have distanced the concerns of the day through watching TV programmes such as *Law and Order* or *CSI* in which a murder is neatly solved in a defined period of time. A wrong is committed, an investigation ensues and a culprit is apprehended and punished. If religion had always supplied a framework for processing guilt, perhaps now it is these cultural products that fill the same space. In this sense, these pre-sleep activities are treatments of conscience, externalisations of guilt and resolution.

It is interesting that these programmes and films frequently make the person who solves the crime the one who was initially suspected. A family member, detective or stranger in town is accused of involvement in the crime, and spends the rest of the narrative effectively demonstrating that it is not they who are guilty but someone else. Closure can take place when guilt has been moved away from the protagonist, and the responsibility for an act of violence situated elsewhere. As Martha Wolfenstein and Nathan Leites observed in their sensational study of film drama, the most frequent motive for crime investigation is to clear oneself of a false charge. There is always some agency – the townsfolk, the local police – that imputes guilt, and the hero has to prove his innocence. Once the guilt is reassigned, then we can sleep.

We could also think here of the way in which children may be sent off to bed as a punishment, although their sentence is more associated with the time spent there *not* sleeping than with sleep itself. A parent might feel outwitted if, after sending off their child, they then find them dozing happily a few minutes later. They are not supposed to be able to sleep! Sleep and a clear conscience once again clash here, and it suggests that there is something linked to guilt that allows us to sleep and something that doesn't.

If we return to the Deri case we discussed earlier, we remember that the patient had a nightly 'wake-hour' at 2 a.m., which the analyst pathologised as a symptom, while for him it was just a normal occurrence. And yet at a certain moment in his analysis, he had the thought that there was a connection between the waking and his childhood history. He remembered that his father would go out every night to see patients, and after his death, when the mother remarried, they would tease her that she had chosen a newspaper editor who would also leave the house every night at the same time. The young man now questioned his mother about the father's sorties, and was told that yes, his father had to set off at 2 a.m. every night to get to the first-aid station where he worked.

The analyst now proposed the interpretation to him that the wake-hour must have some link to the father, and that its very precise time 'kept alive his resentment and his revenge' for having his sleep cruelly interrupted night after night, with the mother failing to protect him from the noise. The patient agreed, and the fury that he had been experiencing in the treatment petered out.

It was not for quite some time now that the wake-hour was mentioned again, yet it would become linked to the central symptom that had brought him to analysis in the first place, his concentration problems in his studies.

He described his attempts to study as a heroic effort to stay awake, and would never fall asleep. When asked why he didn't take short naps if he was so exhausted, he replied, astonished, that he was in fact never tired: 'I always have enough sleep!' And yet he would have to take cold showers, pinch his nose and read aloud what he had to learn. 'I mustn't sleep when I'm supposed to be studying,' he said. 'I always have my eight hours of sound sleep. I should feel terribly guilty if I were to fall asleep in the daytime.' The analyst now asked whether his father could work in the day after his night shifts, and this question brought forth a memory. He had once gone into his father's office and found him asleep on a couch. 'Obviously', he concluded, 'he did not see patients at all.' He had married young and took the night work to contribute to the household expenses, yet his day job was a sham: there was simply no medical practice. As the son's anger emerged in full force now, he voiced his resentment that after his father went out, he was not allowed to join his mother in her bed, as she just wanted to sleep. He had felt completely forsaken.

It now became clear that his sleeping problems had begun after his father's death, but the 2 a.m. waking would only be established after his mother's remarriage, when it was often pointed out that the stepfather left the house at the same time – 2 a.m. – that his father had. Deri comments that 'It was one of his ways of identifying himself with his dead father, a way of conveying to his mother that at least in this respect he was like her husband.' But can't we also see in this another performative dimension, as if he is reminding his family about the father's existence, eclipsed now by the arrival of the new husband? This stepfather, after all, was a well-known newspaper man, author of many books known to the patient's classmates, unlike his less successful father. Suddenly everyone knew about his 'new' father. All the more reason, perhaps, to memorialise the old one.

This situation was complicated by the fact that the boy grew fond of his stepfather, and would do his best to emulate him, especially in writing. He would read stories in his wake-hour and imagine that they were written by his stepfather. He would also plan and write stories himself, while masturbating, and was only sorry that these were mostly never finished because sleep overtook him. All this material did not have any apparent effect on his symptom until some time later in the analysis, when what he perceived as Deri's impatience with him unlocked some new material.

His sense of Deri's lack of time for him evoked not only his father's impatience when he visited his office but also his mother's attitude to his father at night. He now remembered for the first time that his father had actually had no wish to leave at 2 a.m. His mother would become angry and force him to, reprimanding him for his reluctance. Sometimes she would bribe him with kisses or have sex with him as a precondition for his departure. For the boy, this had seemed like a sacrifice, and it was these 'uncanny nights' that lay at the root of his nocturnal symptom. In Deri's construction, 'He was frightened and fascinated, he hated to look on and to listen and he could not bear to go to sleep.' It was after this moment that the patient reported for the first time that he had slept through the night without his wake-hour.

For Deri, the feeling of guilt the young man anticipated were he to fall asleep by day belonged to his wake-hour at night, yet had been displaced so that the night-time hour did not seem symptomatic to him. Hence his surprise that anyone could find it unusual. The guilt had been shifted from the wake-hour to the daytime concern with his studies. Deri is careful to note that in many ways this case is atypical, as so often insomnia does not have such precise causation, in the sense that it is not the bearer of meaning and history. Yet many insomnias do indeed allow this kind of interpretation, fulfilling a specific function at a specific time or, in other cases, gradually accumulating disparate meanings over time, and for this reason are all the more refractory to treatment.

The case, though, is hardly simple, and the young man's night waking was the bearer of several strands of his history that had to be untangled over a long period of time. Although it would be unwise to see all cases of insomnia through the lens of Deri's case, it does suggest something that can clarify and illuminate many other examples. We can remember here the way in which dreams are built, whereby day residues are associated with unconscious trains of thought. The details from our day that are most useful will be those that concern things left undone, what we haven't been able to complete or finish, what we have not dealt with, what we haven't carried through, or what remains unresolved and interrupted: what one eighteenth-century physician called 'the regrets of the day'. These, of course, are basic features of human life, and they tend to gravitate around our points of contact with others, as this is so often where such feelings are generated.

We have not finished a task at work that needs to be seen by others, we have not managed to resolve an interaction with someone else, we have not responded to the demands someone has made on us . . . Now, it is exactly these day residues, so ubiquitous and so easy to conjure, that act like magnets for the unconscious material, which revolves equally around what has not been done, what is left unfinished, what remains unresolved. As Freud observed, the unfinished business of the day shares a 'tenor' with the unsettled conflicts and problems of the unconscious. Sins of omission and unfulfilled duties become magnified, perfect correlates for a guilt at impulses that we may ourselves have repudiated. One guilt thus uses another.

The day residues will touch on everything that is in the order of a debt, what we owe or haven't paid, at a level that goes beyond the empirical debts that we might accumulate. This could be a debt of love, and our sense that we haven't fully paid it, that we have shirked or avoided it: we didn't do what we needed to. Lying awake at night, those who cannot sleep so often describe running through their obligations, what they should have done, how they should have done or do more for their parents, to the point that sleep itself becomes impossible. If sleep is felt as a break, an escape, a suspension of obligations – or as one insomniac put it, 'a checking-out from my obligations' – then, as she continued, 'What right do I have to sleep? How can I forget my obligations?' Sleep would imply a righting of all the wrongs she accused herself of, and in particular, the separation from her parents.

It is perhaps not an accident that we speak of 'sleep debt', an expression that has curiously changed its meaning over the years: at first designating the idea that we spend a third of our lives asleep in order to work off some debt incurred during wakefulness, it now refers to the debt contracted through *not* spending a third of our lives asleep. In Kleitman's first published paper in 1923, he asks the question 'whether eight hours or more of sleep a day really constitutes the minimum penalty for keeping awake the rest of the time', as if wakefulness itself deserves punishment. And to quote once again the striking opening sentence of Gay Luce and Julius Segal's *Insomnia*: 'There is only one sure way to escape insomnia . . . not to be born.' Birth itself introduces a debt, which many people believe can only be paid once they have children.

A patient complained of a persistent and intractable insomnia, and after a great deal of exploration it became clear at what moment it had started. He had been educated at state schools, and after his final exams had won a place at a university abroad. His parents were not in a position to fund this, yet there was nowhere in his country of origin where he could take a course in the subject he wanted to study. His parents supported his choice, and so his mother began night-shift work in order to make the extra money that would be required to let her son pursue his studies. He completed his degree and built a life in the country he had moved to. Now, the sleeping difficulties only began years later, when he learnt that his mother had become unwell.

At one level, what could have been more natural? A son discovers that his mother is sick and he is far away in another country. He can no longer sleep, as he is worrying about her. But this was not actually what had happened. First of all, he was not lying awake consciously thinking about her, and secondly, the insomnia only started some weeks later when he returned to visit her and she made the remark that her health problems had begun during her night-shift work. It was now that the son could no longer sleep. The mother's illness brought out the question of a debt: she had given up her sleep for him, and now, the prospect of her mortality brought home his responsibility. Insomnia was both an identification with his mother – who worked nights for him – and a kind of repayment.

What right, indeed, did he have to sleep? In another case, a casual comment by a mother would mark her daughter's sleep for years to come. At a family gathering she had said during the course of a conversation, 'I didn't sleep for years after the kids were born.' An everyday remark in all its innocence, but for her daughter it carried the signification 'What right then do the children have to sleep?' She was painfully aware of her mother's love of sleep, expressed frequently in her remarks that she craved 'a good night's sleep', and to link this to her birth was to condemn her to a life of sleeplessness.

In another case, a patient described how 'I wake up with a sense of guilt, but I don't know what for, or for whom.' When I quizzed her, no more thoughts were forthcoming: 'How do I know it's guilt? I don't know, but it is.' In a later session, she linked this with the question of her maternity. When she became pregnant, she didn't dare tell her mother, who, many years previously, had once said to her, 'You don't have to have a child.' She had no idea now how her mother would respond to the news: 'There was a guilt there. I was not expected to have a child.' She had interpreted her mother's words as a command, and her own maternity – unconsciously – as a wrongdoing or transgression.

We could also think here of the notion of 'survivor guilt', usually intended to signify the weight of having survived when someone else has died. In the concentration camps, someone might have lived, but their siblings, spouse, children and parents would not have. There is the powerful burden of 'Why not me?', which has been described many times by those who managed to live through the camps. Survivors of other catastrophes have also documented this feeling, from car accidents to terror attacks. Yet isn't it also a feeling that we find in the absence of manifest drama and tragedy, in the bereavements that punctuate every human life?

When someone stops sleeping after a parent has died, however peaceful or predicted the circumstances, there is often this weight of guilt of having survived, of not having been taken instead. There may be the feeling that the parent has given up so much for them, or simply the debt established by being born, but in either case the effects of this debt should not be underestimated, as if there is a certain guilt in staying alive, in surviving, and in separating from those who brought us into the world.

This is in a sense a structural debt, one that cannot be reduced to anything that the person has 'done', yet the very fact of remaining alive may come to take on the status of a guilty act.

Sons and daughters often imagine that they will only gain the independence they seek once they become parents themselves, yet it may well be from this moment onwards that a chronic insomnia is established. It would not be judicious to deny the effects on sleep of having a newborn baby, with all the changes that this introduces to daytime and night-time schedules, but at the same time isn't there also something here in the order of debt? We noted earlier how frequently we hear the vocabulary of punishment: the parent is being kept awake at night as if to be punished, just as an infant's sleep difficulties can so readily be ascribed to one's own deficiencies.

And don't people so often feel guilt at omitting to brush their teeth or remove their make-up for one single night, as if some massive consequence will follow? As one college student put it, 'There is only one thing that will hamper my going to sleep and that is the brushing of my teeth. Not that I worship oral hygiene or that I have a fear of germs, it's just that I hate the guilty feeling of unclean teeth. If I try to sleep without using my toothbrush, it takes longer than usual because I have to concentrate on forgetting about my teeth instead of carelessly relaxing into a pillow.' As bedtime rituals multiply, so the very space for sins of omission becomes sharper.

This idea of an omission is central to one of the most celebrated methods for falling asleep: counting sheep. Although this hardly ever works, it has become synonymous with the process itself of trying to detach from wakefulness. As Wordsworth wrote:

A flock of sheep that leisurely pass by,
One after one; the sound of rain, and bees
Murmuring; the fall of rivers, winds and seas,
Smooth fields, white sheets of water, and pure sky;
I've thought of all by turns; and still I lie
Sleepless.

The poet shows the futility of the exercise, yet its popularity is linked perhaps to the fact that the only real reason to count sheep is to check if one of them has gone missing. The person counting would, of course, be the one responsible for the loss.

In the same way, the rituals we introduce to frame sleep provide miniature dramatisations of reversing this responsibility. Whether it is brushing one's teeth or remembering to swallow a pill or taking the rubbish out, we have a task set for us which we feel we have to carry out. Like the prayers that were once such a staple feature of bedtime, we run through a routine to keep danger at bay and to provide a space that aims to both open and close the possibility of omission, like a nightly treatment of guilt. The effect of neglecting these duties, as the student we quoted above described, shows just how high the hidden stakes of omission may be.

Similarly, just as these tasks present activities that can be completed – unlike most other aspects of our lives – they offer a counterpoint or absolution to what we may experience as the sins of avarice or gluttony: of a 'too much'. Many people lie awake chastising themselves for the pudding, the sugary snack, or second or third cup of coffee or glass of wine that they were guilty of indulging in. As these daily sins are run through and amplified, they come to embody the fault we have perpetrated, a basic responsibility that torments us. The night-time thoughts described here by so many insomniacs oscillate between reproaches for what we omitted or failed to do and what we did but shouldn't have.

These transactions around sleep almost invariably revolve around guilt and blame. As Hartmann observed, receiving a prescription for sleeping pills from a doctor can signify obtaining permission from a parental figure who says, 'It's all right to go to sleep', thus delivering forgiveness for transgressions. And just as Shakespeare's Henry IV longs for sleep to 'steep my senses in forgetfulness', so today's mattresses promise to do this for us. Mattress adverts almost always use a discourse of blame – 'If you aren't sleeping, it's your mattress's fault' – while evoking 'memory foam' or 'mattress memory', as if there is something that needs to be remembered – or of course, forgotten – if we are to sleep properly. At the horizon of all these sleep-related products and processes is an association with conscience and the question of guilt.

Too Guilty to Sleep

As writers and philosophers noticed long before psycho-analysts, there is more than one kind of guilt here. If there is a guilt linked to acts that we have committed, there is also the more structural guilt that such acts may try to localise and absorb. This is the guilt that generates crimes rather than results from them. In Greek tragedy, the protagonist assumes a guilt for actions that fate has already prepared for him. In the *Oresteia*, or Sophocles' Theban plays, characters like Agamemnon and Oedipus are condemned to bear the curse of previous gener-ations. The descendants of Tantalus and of Laius are both agents and victims of a violent curse that haunts their family lineage. Although the dramatists expand and complicate this with questions of individual responsibil-ity, there is a fundamental difference between what the person actually does and the matrix in which their actions are situated.

We see exactly the same distinction in both Freud and Lacan's approaches to the question of guilt. Freud at first saw guilt as a positioning that we might take in relation to early experiences of arousal. At one level, it signifies that we repudiate a sexual drive, perhaps due to a pro-hibition, while at another it is itself a form of sexuality, a way of remaining bound to the drive. Hence the way that many people are unable to enter a sexual relation-ship unless some form of guilt is involved. They seem at times more attached to their guilt than they do to their partner.

Freud thought that we can also experience guilt because of a drive tension, a sense of bodily and psychical urgency and agitation. The push towards satisfaction produces a feeling of guilt, but Freud added that he did not believe in unconscious guilt, as feelings were never unconscious. Their sources could be unconscious, but the sentiments themselves would always be felt consciously at some level. This made him substitute the idea of a need for punishment for that of an unconscious guilt, an observation that chimes with clinical experience, and the fact that patients hardly ever mention insomnia in their first consultations. As for the link between prohibition and guilt, Freud would also abandon this idea, and it is interesting to see how all of his students who studied this question would agree. It might seem obvious that we will feel guilty if we transgress or break the law, yet this is exactly what was contested.

As for the second and more structural form of guilt, Freud found this in transgenerational dynamics. In his just-so story of the origins of society, *Totem and Taboo*, the sons band together to kill the father and gain access to the women of the group, whom the latter had monopolised. But once the deed is done, they are overcome with remorse and now forbid themselves the very women whom their act was intended to deliver. The transmission from one generation to the next in human history of this terrible crime and the remorse that followed it give the parameters of a guilt that does not really result from any action of the individual.

This was the form of guilt that interested Lacan. He distinguished a guilt that resulted from our inscription in kinship systems, a basic debt that we contracted on entering the social world, and a more modern problem of being robbed of this debt. The first form of guilt could be found in classical tragedy, where the heroes and heroines must fulfil their destiny, regardless of the cost to themselves, due to the place they occupy in kinship networks. In a sense, this is a debt of birth, irrevocable and absolute. But a second kind of guilt could arise from having the very idea of destiny removed. Lacan thought that we might feel even more responsible once the appeal to fate is no longer viable, and our preordained pathways are cancelled out.

Indeed, we often find that the sabotaging of a career, a course of study or some other opportunity in life is linked to this question of the loss of a destiny. To be the first person in one's family to go to university, to succeed in business or to rise above a 'station' that they imagine to be their own may produce symptoms that effectively reverse this. Although our culture encourages us to pursue our dreams, and to disregard iniquitous social barriers and prejudices, there can be a heavy price to be paid for this, as if nothing has given the person the right to follow a different trajectory. This is one of the reasons why a depressive phase or some serious error at work may follow what society sees as a 'success'.

As for the first form of guilt, we find a nice example in Christopher Nolan's remake of Erik Skjoldbjaerg's Norwegian thriller Insomnia. A detective accidentally shoots his partner while they are chasing a murderer, an act that is in some ways propitious for him as the dead policeman was about to give evidence against him in an internal affairs investigation. A local officer is charged with writing up the incident, and is happy to sign it off, but the detective insists that she keep the report open. In fact, the shell casing from his own gun would have proven that he and not the murderer had fired the lethal shot. At the end of the film, as he lies dying, she shows him the casing she has now found and offers to cast it away, but he stops her with his last energy. Even though this would risk invalidating his previous arrests and tarnish his name posthumously, it is the inscription of his responsibility that takes precedence.

While he has not been able to sleep throughout the film, it is this last act that allows him to pass into his final slumber. Whereas in the Norwegian original, the officer does in fact set the casing aside, and the detective drives off, Nolan insists on the ontic dimension of guilt: the recognition of what had really happened was more important than the human emotions of relief and the wish to safeguard one's reputation. By insisting that she include the casing in her report, the symbolic order had to be respected, at whatever price. The power of the film lies in this tragic concurrence of two dimensions: the contingent lives of the protagonists and the law of the symbolic universe where guilt cannot be evaded. And once again, the question of guilt is linked to the failure to sleep.

We could also think here of the situation at the end of *The Postman Always Rings Twice*. The protagonist, Frank, and his lover, Cora, murder the latter's husband, making the crime look like a simple car accident. In the complicated chain of blackmail, misunderstanding and error that ensues, almost every single character – even a cat – is guilty of some kind of greater or lesser misdemeanour, and guilt is constantly oscillating from one person to another. Cora finally threatens to implicate Frank in the murder, and in response, he admits to the thought of killing her. Swimming far out to sea just after this scene, she tells him that she is too exhausted to get back to shore, and if he chooses to, he could just leave her there to die. He helps her back, proving his love beyond any doubt. Driving home overjoyed, as they kiss, Frank loses control of the car and Cora is killed.

The accident is mistaken for a crime by the authorities, and Frank is sentenced to death. In the final scene, he desperately questions a priest about whether Cora could have believed him guilty of murdering her in the crash. The district attorney intervenes to explain that he should understand his fate as punishment not for her death but for that of the husband they had murdered, as if justice and divine retribution are finally being served. With this, Frank can accept his sentence. Rather than evading guilt, he can assume it, knowing that he can enter the final sleep only when the record has been set straight. Where in *Insomnia* this record was a human one, in *The Postman* it is abstract and divine.

A counter-example might be found in Margaret Mead's famous descriptions of sleep patterns in Bali. If she came home and found her houseboys asleep, she claimed that this was a sure sign that something had been broken or gone missing. Similarly, in the courthouse, those about to be sentenced on the most serious charges could often be found sleeping soundly on the benches. Although so much of Mead's fieldwork has been challenged, this observation seems to have been accurate, and her findings were replicated many years later in the 1990s. She interpreted these odd siestas as a flight into sleep, as if slumber were an antidote to anxiety, in contrast to the American model of coping with a difficult situation through arousal and vigilance.

But couldn't we see sleep here as what becomes possible only once one's guilty action or trespass has been recognised? Like the shell casing in *Insomnia* or the confession in *The Postman Always Rings Twice*, its inclusion rather than its repression is what allows sleep. There is a big difference, after all, between silently knowing that one has committed a crime or fault, and its social inscription. It is well known clinically that someone who has committed a crime is often able to sleep not after the act but only after the eventual conviction. It is a social recognition of guilt that has an effect on sleep here, and we can wonder what the effects are for those people who have committed a crime yet then managed to evade sentencing or capture. There will often be a second offence now, as if the punishment and, crucially, the recognition of guilt that this involves must be found. When therapy is at times offered to prisoners embarking on a jail term it would thus seem logical to also offer it to those who, on the contrary, have escaped one.

I wonder though how far a talking therapy can go in the receipt and acknowledgement of certain forms of guilt. Although there are indisputably effects here, as guilt is recognised and clarified where it might have been eclipsed, forgotten or foreclosed, there is always the question of its public dimension. How far can a talking therapy go, say, in the case of a soldier who describes his mistaken shooting of an unarmed civilian in a moment of panic and confusion, or of a doctor who remembers having made a clinical error decades previously that resulted in a patient's death? Don't such examples warrant a form of articulation that goes beyond the private space of the consulting room?

Of course, there are forms of public and semi-public space that may respond to this, from a tribunal to a support group to a fellowship, although they are often inaccessible for reasons both social and geographical. If some forms of guilt can certainly be explored, marked and at times attenuated in a talking therapy, there are others that require, in addition, another kind of space. This is not just about a simple fact of admission, but a long work of articulation, in dialogue with others. Admission itself, as Martin Buber beautifully observed of Dostoevsky's Stavrogin, can often be coherent with a crime or a complicity. 'The content of the confession is true, but the act of making it is fictitious,' Buber wrote, so that he 'commits the confession as he commits his crimes'.

—

Can we expect to sleep only once we have a clear conscience? If our unconscious psychical life is full of a sexuality and violence that we would surely repudiate were we to become aware of it, any prospect of a good night's sleep looks bleak. Add to this the guilt and need for punishment that may arise from an unconscious sense of debt and things look even worse. Religious discourse is not to blame here, as we are the harshest judges of ourselves, and we live in a time of merciless and pervasive evaluation. As we have seen, the unconscious fixes on what we have left undone, failed to finish or left incomplete during the day, and inflects these in order to pursue its own aims. Given these conditions, sleep seems increasingly miraculous.

The relatively recent invention of the neat block of eight hours' sleep does not sit well with this. A cartoon in *The Guardian* last year presented a new diagnostic category for the syndrome of believing that we have done everything that we are supposed to do. Sufferers feel that they are on top of things, have managed to complete all required tasks and can cross off every item on their to-do list. Such beliefs are clearly so disconnected from reality that a new diagnostic label is necessary to name them. Although people have made lists for quite a few centuries now, the cartoon brings out the sense of continuous, unrelenting demands that our digital culture makes possible, and the daily sense of exasperation and pressure that this entails.

Impossible to totally sign off, we then receive the instruction to sleep happily for eight hours, waking refreshed and enthusiastic for the day ahead. We must surely treat such imperatives with caution, and recognise what we can and what we can't do. Like many other aspects of modern life, a gap opens up between what a norm tells us to do and our reality, a gap that presents a huge economic opportunity for purveyors of sleep aids, whether in the form of medications and treatments, new mattresses, sleep-tracking apps and devices, or expensive advice from the new sleep experts delivered to banks and large businesses.

The more that the healthy eight-hour block is insisted

upon, the more that pathologies of sleep will be generated as deviations from this norm, and the more pressure put on people to sleep soundly whose lives may not actually permit this. Experiencing sleep as a task to be performed may make it all the more difficult to achieve, and it might help us to recognise that broken, fractured sleep is the rule rather than the exception here. This may well be bad for our health, but the insistence to reach an unattainable ideal of sleep may also be. No one measures what it feels like to strive for a sleep that escapes us, or factors in the effects of the sense of failure that may result.

Sleeping, as we have seen, involves a separation from the demands of others, a distancing from the interpellative side of language and discourse. As we drift into sleep, there will be a time when this function is highlighted, as we either wake suddenly to often nonsensical words or images that seem important to us, or, on the contrary, to those that seem to have no bearing on us. Language either calls us here or releases us. And once we move through this liminal space, we can sleep if our detachment from the interpellative function continues. Finally, on waking, we reconnect with it, and we could even define wakefulness as simply our openness to interpellation. Think of all those scenes in films and TV programmes where someone's name is being called and they do not respond, whether their eyes are open or closed, as if the failure to react to hearing one's name and being asleep are just one and the same thing.

The resemblance of the EEG of wakefulness and that of REM sleep seems no accident here, as interpellation can never be entirely negated during sleep. Dreams help us by disguising and encrypting the desires, traumatic encounters and coercive forces that trouble us, and when this ciphering fails, and we come too close to something unthinkable, we wake up. The mind is constantly busy during sleep, and its operations here have barely begun to be uncovered. The research we have looked at shows that sleep is anything but a natural state; it must be carefully engineered and shaped, and is perpetually vulnerable to disruption, abbreviation and interruption.

We have seen how important the relational aspects of life are for sleep, but perhaps our proximity to other people and their demands means that perfect, untroubled sleep is ultimately in some sense incompatible with human life. Too much is there to wake us up, and one could even go so far as to argue that some form of insomnia is really the baseline of everyday sleeping habits. Language and thought don't just go away at night, and the complex networks of our dependencies continue to have their effects whatever time the clock tells us. If this is the case, what we should expect from sleep changes.

Many people find the idea of biphasic sleep helpful here, so that when they awaken during the night they don't immediately start to panic about missing the eight-hour norm. They realise that they are just doing what human beings have been doing for centuries. Rather than focusing on the idea of going back to sleep, they might choose just to wait out their ninety-minute cycle, to reach the next dip which may make sleep easier. How this time is experienced will depend, of course, on the individual and their own history, and no tracking device or measuring apparatus can tell us what it is; only the words of the person in question. Insomnia, as has often been pointed out, is not lack of sleep but the *complaint* of lack of sleep, and insomniacs, in this sense, need to be listened to.

If the biphasic model can be felt as liberating here, undoing the constraints of consolidated sleep, we might still be wary of the association of sleep with emancipation. Is it an accident, after all, that sleep problems tend to be mentioned so late – if at all – by people in talking therapy? Can't the time spent lying awake be equated, exactly as many insomniacs describe, with a punishment, and the unconscious guilt that can so easily find its correlates in the tasks, duties and interactions that we fail to complete in our waking lives?

The fact that biphasic sleep has probably been around for a long time, and certainly preceded the demand for consolidated sleep, does not make it for all that a natural state. Rather than seeing it as the immutable biological bedrock of the sleep cycle, is it not already marked by the fracture of human subjectivity? Isn't sleep broken not by some natural rhythm but by the splinter of guilt and debt that writers have for centuries situated at the centre of the insomniac's world? Perhaps the 'watching' hour of biphasic sleep was always a symptom of guilt, and it is this that really keeps us awake, something that a sleeping pill can defer but never delete.

Notes

p. 1 Sigmund Freud, *The Interpretation of Dreams* (1899), Standard Edition, Vol. 4, London, Hogarth Press, 1953, p. 229. Facts about sleep, see Herman Regelsberger, *Das Problem des Schlafes*, Berlin, Springer, 1933; Ulrich Ebbecke, 'Physiologie des Schlafes', in L. Adler et al., *Handbuch der normalen und pathologischen Physiologie*, Vol. 17, Berlin, Springer, 1926; Paul Chauchard, *Le Sommeil et les états de sommeil*, Paris, Flammarion, 1947; Otto Marburg, *Der Schlaf*, Berlin, Springer, 1928; and Otto Pötzl, 'Der Schlaf als Behandlungsproblem', in *Der Schlaf*, ed. D. Sarason, Munich, Lehmann, 1929.

p. 3 $76.7 billion, see Patrick Sisson, 'The science (and business) of sleep', *Curbed*, 6 October 2016. Edinburgh University, see Ian Oswald, *Sleep*, Harmondsworth, Penguin, 1966.

p. 5 Thresholds, see Robert Aronowitz, *Making Sense of Illness*, Cambridge University Press, 1998. New research, see Dagfinn Aune et al., 'Fruit and vegetable intake and the risk of cardiovascular disease, total cancer and all-cause mortality – a systematic review and dose-response meta-analysis of prospective studies', *International Journal of Epidemiology*, 46, 2017, pp. 1029–56.

p. 6 Sixteenth-century physician, see Andrew Boorde, 'A compendyous regyment or a dyetary of helthe' (1542), in H. J. Deverson, ed., *Journey into Night*, London, Leslie Frewin, 1966, p. 173. Jon Mooallem, 'The sleep-industrial complex', *New York Times* magazine, 18 November 2007.

p. 7 William Dement, *Some Must Watch While Some Must Sleep*, San Francisco, Freeman, 1972, p. 4. Two American writers, see Robert McGraw and John Oliven, 'Miscellaneous therapies', in Silvano Arieti, ed., *American Handbook of Psychiatry*, 2, New York, Basic Books, 1959, pp. 1442–1582.

p. 8 Matthew Wolf-Meyer, *The Slumbering Masses*, University of Minnesota Press, 2012, p. 147.

p. 9 Study and treatment of apnoea, see Kenton Kroker, *The Sleep of Others and the Transformations of Sleep Research*, University of Toronto Press, 2007. On the rise of apnoea, see ibid., and Tiago Moreira, 'Sleep, health and the dynamics of biomedicine', *Social Science and Medicine*, 63, 2006, pp. 54–63. Insomnia, compare Gay Luce and Julius Segal, *Insomnia*, New York, Doubleday, 1966, with Dieter Riemann et al., 'European guideline for the diagnosis and treatment of insomnia', *Journal of Sleep Research*, 26, 2017, pp. 675–700.

p. 10 Kroker, *The Sleep of Others*, op. cit. Single unit of sleep, see A. Roger Ekirch, *At Day's Close*, New York, Norton, 2005; Benjamin Reiss, *Wild Nights*, New York, Basic Books, 2017; and Wolf-Meyer, *The Slumbering Masses*, op. cit.

p. 11 Nathaniel Kleitman, *Sleep and Wakefulness as Alternating Phases in the Cycle of Existence*, University of Chicago Press, 1939. Meat business, see Nathaniel Kleitman and Theodore Engelmann, 'Sleep characteristics of infants', *Journal of Applied Physiology*, 6, 1953, pp. 269–82. Military, see Eyal Ben-Ari, 'Sleep and night-time combat in contemporary armed forces', in Brigitte Steger and Lodewijk Brunt, eds. *Night-Time and Sleep in Asia and the West*, London, Routledge, 2003, pp. 108–26.

p. 12 Overestimate, see Isabelle Rioux et al., 'Time estimation in chronic insomnia sufferers', *Sleep*, 29, 2006, pp. 486–93; and C. S. Fichten et al., 'Time estimation in good and poor sleepers', *Journal of Behavioral Medicine*, 28, 2005, pp. 537–53. Incommensurable, see Gayle Green, *Insomniac*, University of California Press, 2008, pp. 270–72. Microarousals, see Bernd Feige et al., 'The microstructure of sleep in primary insomnia', *International Journal of Psychophysiology*, 89, 2013, pp. 171–80.

p. 14 Bedtime prayer, see Peter Stearns et al., 'Children's sleep: sketching historical change', *Journal of Social History*, 30, 1996, pp. 345–66.

p. 15 Most prevalent, see Thomas Anders and Pearl Weinstein, 'Sleep and its disorders in infants and children: a review', in Stella Chess and Alexander Thomas, eds., *Annual Progress in Child Psychiatry and Child Development 1973*, New York, Brunner/Mazel, 1974, pp. 377–95.

p. 18 Sleep hygienist, see Matthew Walker, *Why We Sleep*, London, Allen Lane, 2017, pp. 107 and 301.

p. 20 Traffic accidents, see Steven Lockley and Russell Foster, *Sleep*, Oxford University Press, 2012, p. 91. Data now questioned in Rachel Carey and Kiran Sarma, 'Impact of daylight saving time on road traffic collision risk: a systematic review', *BMJ Open*, 7, 2017, e014319.

p. 21 E. P. Thompson, 'Time, work-discipline and industrial capitalism', *Past & Present*, 38, 1967, pp. 56–97; and Vanessa Ogle, *The Global Transformation of Time, 1870–1950*, Harvard University Press, 2015.

p. 22 Walter Benjamin, *The Arcades Project*, Cambridge, Mass., Belknap Press of Harvard University Press, 1999, p. 737.

p. 23 Circadian rhythms, see Russell Foster and Leon Kreitzman, *Rhythms of Life*, London, Profile, 2004. Schedules, see Wolf-Meyer, *The Slumbering Masses*, op. cit., p. 165.

p. 24 Historians, see Ekirch, *At Day's Close*, op. cit. Artificial lighting, see Craig Koslofsky, *Evening's Empire: A History of the Night in Early Modern Europe*, Cambridge University Press, 2011.

p. 26 Basic biology, see Ekirch, *At Day's Close*, op. cit., and 'The modernization of Western sleep: or, does insomnia have a history?', *Past & Present*, 226, 2015, pp. 149–92.

p. 27 Children of the night, see Sasha Handley, *Sleep in Early Modern England*, Yale University Press, 2016, p. 151.

p. 28 Thomas Wehr, 'In short photoperiods, human sleep is biphasic', *Journal of Sleep Research*, 1, 1992, pp. 103–7. Controversy, see discussion in Reiss, *Wild Nights*, op. cit., pp. 34–7.

p. 30 Paul Glennie and Nigel Thrift, *Shaping the Day: A History of Timekeeping in England and Wales 1300–1800*, Oxford University Press, 2009, and the critique by Jonathan Martineau, 'Making sense of the history of clock time, reflections on Glennie and Thrift's *Shaping the Day*', *Time & Society*, 26, 2017, pp. 305–20.

p. 31 Jonathan Crary, *24/7: Late Capitalism and the Ends of Sleep*, London, Verso, 2013. Standardised, see Ogle, *The Global Transformation of Time*, op. cit.; and Kevin Birth, 'Time and the biological consequences of globalization', *Current Anthropology*, 48, 2007, pp. 215–36.

p. 32 Henry Ford, *My Life and Work* (1922), London, Heinemann, 1931, p. 24.

p. 33 China, see Steger and Brunt, eds. *Night-Time and Sleep in Asia and the West*, op. cit.

p. 34 Napping, see Brigitte Steger, 'Negotiating sleep patterns in Japan', in ibid., pp. 65–86; and Simon Williams et al., 'Medicalisation or customisation? Sleep, enterprise and enhancement in the 24/7 society', *Social Science and Medicine*, 79, 2013, pp. 40–47.

p. 36 Bedtime classic, see Margaret Wise Brown, *Goodnight Moon*, New York, Harper, 1947.

p. 37 Surveys, see for example First Psychology Scotland, *The Impact of Technology on Work/Life Balance and Wellbeing*, Edinburgh, 2015; Judy Wajcman et al., 'Families without borders: mobile phone connectedness and work-home divisions', *Sociology*, 42, 2008, pp. 635–52; and Judy Wajcman et al., 'The impact of the mobile phone on work/life balance', *AMTA*, June 2007. Erving Goffman, *Asylums*, New York, Doubleday, 1961.

p. 39 Chloe Aridjis, 'Insomnia begins in the cradle: creating a narrative', presented at CFAR conference, London, 8 July 2017.

p. 43 Ernest Hartmann, *The Sleeping Pill*, Yale University Press, 1978, p. 1. Walker, *Why We Sleep*, op. cit., pp. 7 and 26.

p. 44 Luce and Segal, *Insomnia*, op. cit. Emotion, see Ruth Leys, 'How did fear become a scientific object and what kind of object is it?', *Representations*, 110, 2010, pp. 66–104.

p. 46 Olympic gold medallists, see Ruth Leys, *From Guilt to Shame: Auschwitz and After*, Princeton University Press, 2007, p. 142.

p. 47 Market-based societies, see Nikolas Rose, *Governing the Soul*, London, Routledge, 1990. Two simple rules, see Walker, *Why We Sleep*, op. cit., pp. 246–7.

p. 49 Frances Deri, 'Symposium on neurotic disturbances of sleep', *International Journal of Psychoanalysis*, 23, 1942, pp. 49–68.

p. 50 The term 'insomnia', see Ekirch, 'The modernization of Western sleep: or, does insomnia have a history?', op. cit.; Eluned Summers-Bremner, *Insomnia: A Cultural History*, London, Reaktion Books, 2008; and Lee Scrivner, *Becoming Insomniac*, New York, Palgrave Macmillan, 2014.

p. 51 Annihilation, see Scrivner, *Becoming Insomniac*, op. cit., pp. 18 and 169. Sleeplessness, *British Medical Journal*, September 1984, p. 719 quoted in Karen Beth Strovas, 'The vampire's night light: artificial light, hypnagogia and quality of sleep in *Dracula*', *Critical Survey*, 27, 2015, pp. 50–66.

p. 53 Georgie Byng, Hampstead Theatre, 18 March 2018.

p. 54 Édouard Claparède, 'Esquisse d'une théorie biologique du sommeil', *Archives de Psychologie*, 4, 1905, pp. 245–359. See also Henri Piéron, *Le Problème Physiologique du sommeil*, Paris, Masson, 1913; and R. D. Gillespie, *Sleep and the Treatment of its Disorders*, London, Baillière, Tindall & Cox, 1929.

p. 55 Immune functioning, see M. R. Opp, 'Cytokines and sleep', *Sleep Medicine Reviews*, 9, 2005, pp. 355–64; M. R. Opp and J. M. Krueger, 'Sleep and immunity: a growing field with clinical impact', *Brain, Behavior, and Immunity*, 47, 2015, pp. 1–3; Sarah Geiger et al., 'Chrono-immunology: progress and challenges in understanding links between the circadian and immune systems', *Immunology*, 146, 2015, pp. 349–58; and Brice Faraut et al., 'Immune, inflammatory and cardiovascular consequences of sleep restriction and recovery', *Sleep Medicine Reviews*, 16, 2012, pp. 137–49.

p. 56 Eugene Aserinsky, 'The discovery of REM sleep', *Journal of the History of the Neurosciences*, 5, 1996, pp. 213–27. Aserinsky downplayed other researchers before him who recognised REM, claiming that they must have been observing slow eye movements and not rapid ones. He quotes George Trumbull Ladd's 1892 paper, 'Contribution to the Psychology of Visual Dreams', *Mind*, 1, 1892, pp. 299–304, that the 'eyeballs move gently in their sockets', yet Ladd is quite explicit in referring to 'rapid movement', and he also makes the scanning hypothesis in this paper. Edmund Jacobson, *You Can Sleep Well*, New York, Whittlesey House, 1938, p. 264, notes that dreaming is signalled by eye movement and can be detected by EEG, as well as differentiating two different kinds of sleep. Ian Oswald, *Sleeping and Waking*, Amsterdam, Elsevier, 1962, p. 35; David Metcalf et al., 'Ontogenesis of spontaneous K-complexes', *Psychophysiology*, 8, 1971, pp. 340–47; C. H. Bastien et al., 'EEG characteristics prior to and following the evoked K-complex', *Canadian Journal of Experimental Psychology*, 54, 2000, pp. 255–65; Birendra Mallick and Shojiro Inoué, eds., *Rapid Eye Movement Sleep*, New York, Marcel Dekker, 1999.

p. 58 Newborns, see Carole Marcus et al., eds., *Sleep in Children*, 2nd edn, New York, Informa, 2008.

p. 60 Giuseppe Moruzzi and Horace Magoun, 'Brain stem reticular formation and activation of the EEG', *Electroencephalography and Clinical Neurophysiology*, 1, 1949, pp. 455–73; Wilse Webb, ed., *Sleep: An Active Process*, Glenview, Ill, Scott, Foresman and Company, 1973. Motility cycle, see Eugene Aserinsky and Nathaniel Kleitman, 'Regularly occurring periods of eye motility, and concomitant phenomena, during sleep', *Science*, 118, 1953, pp. 273–4.

p. 61 Breakthrough, see Dement, *Some Must Watch While Some Must Sleep*, op. cit., p. 25.

p. 62 Zelda Teplitz, 'An electroencephalographic study of dreams and sleep', Masters Thesis, University of Chicago, 1943. Reporter, see Kroker, *The Sleep of Others*, op. cit., p. 286.

p. 63 Colourful images, see Louise Whiteley, 'Resisting the revelatory scanner? Critical engagements with fMRI in popular media', *BioSocieties*, 7, 2012, pp. 245–72; Sarah de

Rijcke and Anne Beaulieu, 'Networked neuroscience: brain scans and visual knowing at the intersection of atlases and databases', in Catelijne Coopmans et al., eds., *Representation in Scientific Practice Revisited*, Cambridge, Mass., MIT Press, 2014, pp. 131–52; Anne Beaulieu, 'Images are not the (only) truth: brain mapping, visual knowledge and iconoclasm', *Science, Technology, & Human Values*, 27, 2002, pp. 53–86; and Kelly Joyce, *Magnetic Appeal: MRI and the Myth of Transparency*, Cornell University Press, 2008.

p. 66 Russian research, see M. P. Denisova and N. L. Figurin, 'Periodic occurrences in the sleep of children', *New Work in Reflexology and Physiology of the Nervous System*, Vol. 2, State Psychoneurological Academy and State Reflexology Institute of Brain Research, Leningrad, 1926, pp. 338–45.

p. 67 Consolidation of memories, see G. E. Müller and A. Pilzecker, 'Experimentelle Beiträge zur Lehre vom Gedächtniss', *Zeitschrift für Psychologie und Psychologie der Sinnesorgane*, Supplement 1, Leipzig, Barth, 1900. Electrical current, compare Walker, *Why We Sleep*, op. cit., pp. 111 and 114, with the more balanced review in Larry Squire et al., 'Memory consolidation', *Cold Spring Harbor Perspectives in Biology*, 7, 2015, a021766 and H. Freyja Ólafsdóttir et al., 'The role of hippocampal replay in memory and planning', *Current Biology*, 28, 2018, R37–R50. See also Robert Vertes and Kathleen Eastman, 'The case against memory consolidation in REM sleep', *Behavioral and Brain Sciences*, 23, 2000, pp. 867–76; Robert Vertes and J. M. Siegel, 'Time for the sleep community to take a critical look at the purported role of sleep in memory processing', *Sleep*, 28, 2005, pp. 1228–9; and Marcos Frank and Joel Benington, 'The role of sleep in memory consolidation and brain plasticity: dream or reality?', *The Neuroscientist*, 12, 2006, pp. 1–12.

p. 69 Jocelyn Small, *Wax Tablets of the Mind: Cognitive Studies of Memory and Literacy in Classical Antiquity*, London, Routledge, 1997; and Frances Yates, *The Art of Memory*, University of Chicago Press, 1966. See also Claudia Infurchia, *La Mémoire entre neurosciences et psychanalyse*, Toulouse, Érès, 2014.

p. 73 Leys, *From Guilt to Shame*, op. cit.

p. 74 Primo Levi, *The Drowned and the Saved*, New York, Simon and Schuster, 1989, p. 38, quoted in Leys, *From Guilt to Shame*, op. cit.

p. 75 Sleep hygienist, see Walker, *Why We Sleep*, op. cit., pp. 122–3.

p. 76 Rewriting, see Frederic Bartlett, *Remembering*, Cambridge University Press, 1932.

p. 77 Leslie Dwyer and Degung Santikarma, 'Posttraumatic politics: violence, memory, and biomedical discourse in Bali', in Laurence Kirmayer et al., eds. *Understanding Trauma*, Cambridge University Press, 2007, pp. 403–32. Culling, see Francis Crick and Graeme Mitchison, 'The function of dream sleep', *Nature*, 304, 1983, pp. 111–14; Walker, *Why We Sleep*, op. cit., pp. 45, 120 and 217; and G. Tononi and C. Cirelli, 'Sleep and the price of plasticity', *Neuron*, 81, 2014, pp. 12–34.

p. 80 Herman Witkin and Helen Lewis, 'The relation of experimentally induced presleep experiences to dreams', *Journal of the American Psychoanalytic Association*, 13, 1965, pp. 819–49, and 'Presleep experiences and dreams', in Herman Witkin and Helen Lewis, eds., *Experimental Studies of Dreaming*, New York, Random House, 1967, pp. 148–201.

p. 82 Bali, see Dwyer and Santikarma, 'Posttraumatic politics', op. cit. War trauma, see K. C. Hyams et al., 'War syndromes and their evaluation: from the US Civil War to the Persian Gulf War', *Annals of Internal Medicine*, 125, 1996, pp. 398–405; Ruth Leys, *Trauma: A Genealogy*, University of Chicago Press, 2000; and Allan Young, *The Harmony of Illusions: Inventing Post-Traumatic Stress Disorder*, Princeton University Press, 1995.

p. 84 Abduction, see R. J. McNally et al., 'Psychophysiological responding during script-driven imagery in people reporting abduction by space aliens', *Psychological Science*, 15, 2004, pp. 493–7. Borrowed memory, see Darian Leader, *The New Black: Mourning, Melancholia and Depression*, London, Hamish Hamilton, 2008, pp. 75–84.

p. 85 Joseph Robertson can be heard on StoryCorps Oral History Project, youtube.com/watch?v=trmGomgrkM8.

p. 87 Adaptation to society, see P. Lavie and H. Kaminer, 'Dreams that poison sleep: dreaming in Holocaust survivors', *Dreaming*, 1, 1991, pp. 11–22. Individual psychotherapy, see Hugo Schwerdtner, in Meeting of the Vienna Psychoanalytic Society, 23 October 1907, in Herman Nunberg and Ernst Federn, eds., *Minutes of the Vienna Psychoanalytic Society*, 1, New York, International Universities Press, 1962, p. 219.

p. 90 Scanning, see W. Dement and N. Kleitman, 'The relation of eye movements during sleep to dream activity: an objective method for the study of dreaming', *Journal of Experimental Psychology*, 53, 1957, pp. 339–46; L. Jacobs et al., 'Are the eye movements of dreaming sleep related to the visual images of dreams?', *Psychophysiology*, 9, 1972, pp. 393–401; and John Herman et al., 'Evidence for a directional correspondence between eye movements and dream imagery in REM sleep', *Sleep*, 7, 1984, pp. 52–63. Lively dance, Dement, *Some Must Watch While Some Must Sleep*, op. cit.

p. 91 Growth and plasticity, see S. N. Graven and J. V. Browne, 'Sleep and brain development: the critical role of sleep in fetal and early neonatal brain development', *Newborn and Infant Nursing Reviews*, 8, 2008, pp. 173–9.

p. 92 Susan Weiner and Howard Ehrlichman, 'Ocular motility and cognitive process', *Cognition*, 4, 1976, pp. 31–43. Trying to suppress, see J. Antrobus et al., 'Eye movements accompanying daydreaming, visual imagery, and thought suppression', *Journal of Abnormal Psychology*, 69, 1964, pp. 244–52.

p. 93 Dream recall, see Donald Goodenough, 'Dream recall: history and current status of the field', in Arthur Arkin et al., eds., *The Mind in Sleep*, Hillsdale, Lawrence Erlbaum, 1978, pp. 113–42; John Herman et al., 'The problem of NREM dream recall re-examined', in ibid., pp. 59–96; Edward Wolpert, 'Two classes of factors affecting dream recall', *Journal of the American Psychoanalytic Association*, 20, 1972, pp. 45–58; and the review in Milton Kramer, *The Dream Experience*, New York, Routledge, 2012, pp. 33–50.

p. 94 Financial incentives, see Allan Rechtschaffen and Paul Verdone, 'Amount of dreaming: effect of incentive, adaptation to laboratory, and individual differences', *Perceptual and Motor Skills*, 19, 1964, pp. 947–58. Covert REM, see Tore Nielsen, 'A review of mentation in REM and NREM sleep: "covert" REM sleep as a possible reconciliation of two opposing models', in Edward Pace-Schott et al., eds., *Sleep and Dreaming*, Cambridge University Press, 2003, pp. 59–74. Joe Kamiya had apparently explored REM against a background of slow eye movement in 'Slow and rapid eye movements during Stage 1 sleep', *Association for the Psychophysiological Study of Sleep*, 1963 (unpublished). To use REM as a measure, the meaning of dreaming had indeed changed, as Dement noticed: 'Psychophysiology of Sleep and Dreams', in Silvano Arieti, ed., *American Handbook of Psychiatry*, 3, New York, Basic Books, 1966, pp. 290–32. Other variables, see Donald Goodenough, 'Some recent studies of dream recall', in Witkin and Lewis, eds., *Experimental Studies of Dreaming*, op. cit., pp. 128–47; and Arthur Shapiro et al., 'Gradual arousal from sleep: a determinant of thinking reports', *Psychosomatic Medicine*, 27, 1965, pp. 342–9.

p. 95 Middle ear, see M. A. Pessah and H. P. Roffwarg, 'Spontaneous middle ear muscle activity in man: a rapid eye movement sleep phenomenon', *Science*, 178, 1972, pp. 773–6; and H. Roffwarg et al., 'The middle ear muscles: predictability of their phasic activity in REM sleep from dream material', *Sleep Research*, 4, 1975, p. 165.

p. 96 Motif, see Allan Rechtschaffen et al., 'Interrelatedness of mental activity during sleep', *Archives of General Psychiatry*, 9, 1963, pp. 536–47. Hypnotised, see Arthur Arkin et al., 'Post-hypnotically stimulated sleep-talking', *Journal of Nervous and Mental Disease*, 142, 1966, pp. 293–309. David Foulkes, 'Dream reports from different stages of sleep', *Journal of Abnormal and Social Psychology*, 65, 1962, pp. 14–25; and the review in David Foulkes, 'Dream Research: 1953–1993', *Sleep*, 19, 1996, pp. 609–24. See also Corrado Cavallero et al., 'Slow wave sleep dreaming', *Sleep*, 15, 1992, pp. 562–6. Poor cousin, see R. T. Pivik, 'Tonic states and phasic events in relation to sleep mentation', in Arkin et al., eds., *The Mind in Sleep*, op. cit. pp. 245–71.

p. 97 Relation between REM and NREM, see the suggestive discussion in Joel Benington, 'Why we believe what we believe about REM-sleep regulation', in Mallick and Inoué, eds., *Rapid Eye Movement Sleep*, op. cit., pp. 393–401.

p. 98 GSR storms, see Oswald, *Sleep*, op. cit., p. 72.

p. 99 Doctor fell asleep, see Morton Reiser, 'Reflections on interpretation of psychophysiologic experiments', *Psychosomatic Medicine*, 23, 1961, pp. 430–39. Dement and Kleitman described movements of the fingers in their original report 'Cyclic variations of EEG during sleep and their relation to eye movements, body motility, and dreaming', *Electroencephalography and Clinical Neurophysiology*, 9, 1957, pp. 673–90, and a lot of activity can be recorded by refining measurement techniques. See Bill Baldridge et al., 'The concurrence of fine muscle activity and rapid eye movements during sleep', *Psychosomatic Medicine*, 27, 1965, pp. 19–26. Jacobson, *You Can Sleep Well*, op. cit., used arm muscle voltage and activity to index dreaming (pp. 199 and 264).

p. 100 Puppet, see Oswald, *Sleeping and Waking*, op. cit., p. 199. Missed REM, see for example L. Palm et al., 'Sleep and wakefulness in normal preadolescent children', *Sleep*, 12, 1989, pp. 299–308, and I. Karacan et al., 'Erection cycle during sleep in relation to dream anxiety', *Archives of General Psychiatry*, 15, 1966, pp. 183–9. Different functions, see Thomas Anders, 'An overview of recent sleep and dream research', *Psychoanalysis and Contemporary Science*, 3, 1974, pp. 449–69.

p. 102 Sigmund Freud, *The Interpretation of Dreams*, Standard Edition, Vol. 5, London, Hogarth Press, 1953, p. 553.

p. 104 Ancel Keys et al., *The Biology of Human Starvation*, University of Minnesota Press, 1950. Anchovy-induced dream, see Freud, *The Interpretation of Dreams*, op. cit., Vol. 4, pp. 123–4. On desire and wish, see Pierre Bruno, *Qu'est-ce que rêver?*, Toulouse, Érès , 2017. See also the review of analytic work on dreams in Kramer, *The Dream Experience*, op. cit.

p. 105 Dement, *Some Must Watch While Some Must Sleep*, op. cit., p. 53.

p. 106 Freud, *The Interpretation of Dreams*, op. cit., Vol. 5, p. 581.

p. 107 Walker, *Why We Sleep*, op. cit., p. 202.

p. 108 Exaggerated respect, see Sigmund Freud, 'Remarks on the Theory and Practice of Dream-Interpretation' (1923), in *The Ego and the Id and Other Works*, Standard Edition, Vol. 19, London, Hogarth, 1961, p. 112.

p. 109 Lemon, see Edmund Bergler, 'An enquiry into the "material phenomenon"', *International Journal of Psychoanalysis*, 16, 1935, pp. 203–18.

p. 113 A father, Freud, *The Interpretation of Dreams*, op. cit., Vol. 5, pp. 509–11.

p. 114 Jacques Lacan, *The Seminar XI: The Four Fundamental Concepts of Psychoanalysis* (1964), ed. J.-A. Miller, London, Hogarth, 1977, pp. 57–60.

p. 116 Never fully awake, Lawrence Kubie, 'The concept of dream deprivation: a critical analysis', *Psychosomatic Medicine*, 24, 1962, pp. 62–5; and Lawrence Kubie, in Heinz von Foerster, ed., *Cybernetics: Transactions of the Eighth Conference, March 15–16, 1951*, New York, Josiah Macy, Jr. Foundation, 1952, p. 94. Several claims, see Ekkehard Othmer et al., 'Encephalic cycles during sleep and wakefulness in humans: a 24 hour pattern', *Science*, 164, 1969, pp. 447–9; and Gordon Globus, 'Rapid eye movement cycle in real time', *Archives of General Psychiatry*, 15, 1966, pp. 654–9. Norbert Wiener, see von Foerster, ed., *Cybernetics*, op. cit., p. 92. Eyes open, see A. Fuchs and F. C. Wu, 'Sleep with half-open eyes (physiologic lagophthalmus)', *American Journal of Ophthalmology*, 31, 1948, pp. 717–20.

p. 117 150-watt bulb, see Oswald, *Sleeping and Waking*, op. cit., p. 46. Contact with reality, see David Foulkes and S. Fleischer, 'Mental activity in relaxed wakefulness', *Journal of Abnormal Psychology*, 84, 1975, pp. 66–75. Scientific lecture, see Martin Grotjahn, 'The process of awakening', *The Psychoanalytic Review*, 29, 1942, pp. 1–19.

p. 118 Viktor Frankl, *Man's Search for Meaning*, New York, Washington Square Press, 1963, p. 45.

p. 119 Dickens, see John Cosnett, 'Charles Dickens and Sleep Disorders', *The Dickensian*, 93, 1997, pp. 200–204. Scrivner, *Becoming Insomniac*, op. cit., p. 115.

p. 120 Joseph Collins, *Sleep and the Sleepless*, New York, Sturgis & Walton, 1912.

p. 121 Vincent Dachy, see Buster V. Dachy, *The Crumpled Envelope*, London, Ma Bibliothèque, 2017.

p. 122 Interpellate, see Darian Leader, 'The voice as psychoanalytic object', *Analysis*, 12, 2003, pp. 70–82; and Darian Leader, *What is Madness?*, London, Hamish Hamilton, 2011, pp. 156–69.

p. 123 Stab in the heart, see Eugen Kogon, *The Theory and Practice of Hell*, New York, Farrar, Straus and Cudahy, 1950, p. 78. Ruth Weir, *Language in the Crib*, The Hague, Mouton, 1962.

p. 124 Uninterruptedly, see Sigmund Freud, *Introductory Lectures on Psycho-Analysis* (1915–16), Standard Edition, Vol. 15, London, Hogarth, 1961, p. 88. Jan Linschoten, 'On falling asleep' (1952), in J. J. Kockelmans, ed., *Phenomenological Psychology*, Vol. 103, Dordrecht, Springer, 1987 pp. 79–117.

p. 125 Nocturnal phenomenon, see Andreas Mavromatis, *Hypnagogia*, London, Routledge & Kegan Paul, 1987.

p. 126 Not being addressed, see Emil Froeschels, 'A peculiar intermediary state between waking and sleep', *Journal of Clinical Psychopathology*, 7, 1946, pp. 825–33. Spectacle, see H. Fischgold and S. Safar, 'États de demi-sommeil et images hypnagogiques', in Pierre Wertheimer, ed., *Rêve et conscience*, Paris, PUF, 1968, pp. 187–98; Robert Ogilvie,

'The process of falling asleep', *Sleep Medicine Reviews*, 5, 2001, pp. 247–70.

p. 128 Simon Williams, *Sleep and Society*, London, Routledge, 2005, p. 69. Maurice Merleau-Ponty, *The Phenomenology of Perception* (1945), London, Routledge & Kegan Paul, 1962, pp. 189–90.

p. 129 Proximity, see M. Mirmiran and S. Lunshof, 'Perinatal development of human circadian rhythms', *Progress in Brain Research*, 111, 1996, pp. 217–26; and S. Lunshof et al., 'Fetal and maternal diurnal rhythms during the third trimester of normal pregnancy: outcomes of computerized analysis of continuous 24-hour fetal heart rate recordings', *American Journal of Obstetrics and Gynecology*, 178, 1998, pp. 247–54. Baby's adaptation, see for example K. Nishihara et al., 'The development of infants' circadian rest–activity rhythm and mothers' rhythm', *Physiology & Behavior*, 77, 2002, pp. 91–8; S. Y. Tsai et al., 'Mother–infant activity synchrony as a correlate of the emergence of circadian rhythm', *Biological Research for Nursing*, 13, 2011, pp. 80–88; and Karen Thomas et al., 'Maternal and infant activity: analytic approaches for the study of circadian rhythm', *Infant Behavior & Development*, 41, 2015, pp. 80–87.

p. 130 Unaware, see B. L. Goodlin-Jones et al., 'Night waking, sleep–wake organization, and self-soothing in the first year of life', *Journal of Developmental and Behavioral Pediatrics*, 22, 2001, pp. 226–33; and L. Tikotzky and A. Sadeh, 'Sleep patterns and sleep disruptions in kindergarten children', *Journal of Clinical Child Psychology*, 30, 2001, pp. 581–91. Kleitman and Engelmann, 'Sleep characteristics of infants', op. cit.; Theodor Hellbrügge, 'Ontogénèse des rythmes circardiairies chez l'enfant', in Julian de Ajuriaguerra, ed., *Cycles biologiques et psychiatrie*, Geneva, Georg, 1968, pp. 159–83; Hellbrügge, 'The development of circadian rhythms in infants', *Cold Spring Harbor Symposia on Quantitative Biology*, 25, 1960, pp. 311–23; Theodor Hellbrügge, 'The development of circadian and ultradian rhythms of premature and full-term infants', in Lawrence Scheving, et al., eds., *Chronobiology*, Tokyo, Shoin, 1974, pp. 339–41; Claire Beugnet-Lambert, 'Les rythmes de l'enfant de la naissance à l'adolescence', in Pierre Leconte et al., eds., *Chronopsychologie: rythmes et activités humaines*, Presses Universitaires de Lille, 1988, pp. 133–59; S. Coons and C. Guilleminault, 'Development of sleep–wake patterns and non-rapid eye movement sleep stages during the first six months of life in normal infants', *Pediatrics*, 69, 1982, pp. 793–8. Feeding, see Eugene Aserinsky and Nathaniel Kleitman, 'A motility cycle in sleeping infants as manifested by ocular and gross bodily activity', *Journal of Applied Physiology*, 8, 1955, pp. 11–18. Rest–activity cycle, see Nathaniel Kleitman, 'Basic rest–activity cycle – 22 years later', *Sleep*, 5, 1982, pp. 311–17.

p. 131 Sanford Gifford, 'Sleep, time, and the early ego', *Journal of the American Psychoanalytic Association*, 8, 1960, pp. 5–42; and Sanford Gifford, 'The prisoner of time', *Annual of Psychoanalysis*, 8, 1980, pp. 131–54. Number of feeds, see T. Moore and L. Ucko, 'Night waking in early infancy: Part I', *Archives of Disease in Childhood*, 32, 1957, pp. 333–42.

p. 132 Anticipate, see Marshall Haith et al., 'Expectation and anticipation of dynamic visual events by 3.5-month-old babies', *Child Development*, 59, 1988, pp. 467–79.

p. 133 René Spitz, 'Some early prototypes of ego defenses', *Journal of the American Psychoanalytic Association*, 9, 1961, pp. 626–51; René Spitz et al., 'Further prototypes of ego formation', *Psychoanalytic Study of the Child*, 25, 1970, pp. 417–41; René Spitz, 'Relevancy of direct infant observation',

Psychoanalytic Study of the Child, 5, 1950, pp. 66–73. Eye movements, see Joan Lynch and Eugene Aserinsky, 'Developmental changes of oculomotor characteristics in infants when awake and in the "active state of sleep"', *Behavioural and Brain Research*, 20, 1986, pp. 175–83; and Eugene Aserinsky et al., 'Comparison of eye motion in wakefulness and REM sleep', *Psychophysiology*, 22, 1985, pp. 1–10. World Health Organization report, see A. Kahn, et al., 'Sleep characteristics and sleep deprivation in infants, children and adolescents', in *WHO Technical Meeting on Sleep and Health*, Bonn: WHO Regional Office for Europe, 2004, pp. 38–61.

p. 134 Synonymous with feeding problems, see Robert Debré and Alice Doumic, *Le Sommeil de l'enfant*, Paris, PUF, 1959, p. 77. Harshly, see Naomi Ragins and Joseph Schachter, 'A study of sleep behavior in two-year-old children', *Journal of the American Academy of Child Psychiatry*, 10, 1971, pp. 464–80.

p. 136 Hunger contractions, see R. E. Scantlebury et al., 'The effect of normal and hypnotically induced dreams on the gastric hunger movements of man', *Journal of Applied Psychology*, 26, 1942, pp. 682–91. Roy Whitman, 'Remembering and forgetting dreams in psychoanalysis', *Journal of the American Psychoanalytic Association*, 11, 1963, pp. 752–74; and Whitman et al., 'The physiology, psychology, and utilization of dreams', *American Journal of Psychiatry*, 124, 1967, pp. 287–302.

p. 137 Banana cream pie, see Dement, *Some Must Watch While Some Must Sleep*, op. cit., p. 65. The other model, see Jacques Lacan, *Le Séminaire, Livre IV: La Relation d'objet* (1956–7), ed. J.-A. Miller, Paris, Seuil, 1994, pp. 181–3.

p. 138 Hartmann, *The Sleeping Pill*, op. cit., p. 132.

p. 143 Ronald Harper et al., 'Effects of feeding on state and cardiac regulation in the infant', *Developmental Psychobiology*, 10, 1977, pp. 507–17. See also Leconte et al., *Chronopsychologie*, op. cit. For a conflicting view, see P. Salzarulo et al., 'Sleep patterns in infants under continuous feeding from birth', *Electroencephalography and Clinical Neurophysiology*, 49, 1980, pp. 330–36.

p. 144 Abruptly hospitalised, see Avi Sadeh, *Sleeping Like a Baby*, Yale University Press, 2001, p. 65. Circumcised, see R. Emde et al., 'Stress and neonatal sleep', *Psychosomatic Medicine*, 33, 1971, pp. 491–7.

p. 145 Popular methods, see Christina Hardyment, *Dream Babies: Child Care from Locke to Spock*, London, Cape, 1983. Air raids, see Tom Harrisson, 'Obscure nervous effects of air raids', *British Medical Journal*, April 1941, pp. 573–4. Oswald, *Sleeping and Waking*, op. cit., p. 158. Ethologists, see Nikolaas Tinbergen, *The Study of Instinct*, 2nd edn, Oxford, Clarendon Press, 1969, p. 210. Spitz et al., 'Further prototypes of ego formation', op. cit.

p. 148 Private sleeping, see Oskar Jenni and Bonnie O'Connor, 'Children's sleep: an interplay between culture and biology', *Pediatrics*, 115, 2005, pp. 204–16; and Stearns et al., 'Children's sleep: sketching historical change', op. cit. Anna Freud, *Normality and Pathology in Childhood*, London, Hogarth, 1965.

p. 149 Isabel Paret, 'Night waking and its relation to mother–infant interactions in nine-month-old infants', in Justin Call et al., eds., *Frontiers of Infant Psychiatry*, New York, Basic Books, 1983, pp. 171–7; M. M. Burnham et al., 'Nighttime sleep–wake patterns and self-soothing from birth to one year of age: a longitudinal intervention study', *Journal of Child Psychology and Psychiatry*, 43, 2002, pp. 713–25.

p. 153 Mark Kanzer, 'The communicative function of the dream', *International Journal of Psychoanalysis*, 36, 1955, pp. 260–6. Mammoth Cave, see footage and newspaper accounts on web; and Matthew Wolf-Meyer, 'Where have all our naps gone? Or Nathaniel Kleitman, the consolidation of sleep, and the historiography of emergence', *Anthropology of Consciousness*, 24, 2013, pp. 96–116. Bizarrely, in a late paper, Kleitman actually cites the frequency of 'Thou shalt not' in the Ten Commandments to explain cortical inhibition in sleep: Kleitman, 'Basic rest–activity cycle – 22 years later', op. cit., pp. 311–17.

p. 155 Discussion and examples of solitary confinement, see Gifford, 'The prisoner of time', op. cit., pp. 131–54; Paul Fraisse et al., 'Le rythme veille-sommeil et l'estimation du temps', in Julian de Ajuriaguerra, ed., *Cycles biologiques et psychiatrie*, op. cit., pp. 257–65; Edith Bone, *Seven Years Solitary*, London, Hamish Hamilton, 1957, p. 115; P. M. van Wulfften Palthe, 'Time sense in isolation', *Psychiatria, Neurologia, Neurochirurgia*, 71, 1968, pp. 221–41; and J. A. Vernon and T. E. McGill, 'Time estimations during sensory deprivation', *Journal of General Psychology*, 69, 1963, pp. 11–18. Michel Siffre, *Beyond Time*, London, Chatto & Windus, 1965.

p. 157 Menninger Clinic, see J. Cotter Hirschberg, 'Parental anxieties accompanying sleep disturbance in young children', *Bulletin of the Menninger Clinic*, 21, 1957, pp. 129–39. See also *The Nervous Child*, 8, 1949 issue on sleep disturbances in children.

p. 158 Marie Darrieussecq, 'Darling insomnia', paper given at CFAR conference, London, 8 July 2017.

p. 159 Being punished, quoted in Green, *Insomniac*, op. cit., p. 1.

p. 161 Devotional texts, see Handley, *Sleep in Early Modern England*, op. cit. Purification, see Jean Delumeau, *Sin and Fear:*

The Emergence of a Western Guilt Culture, 13th–18th Centuries, New York, St Martin's Press, 1990.

p. 162 Thomas Nashe, *The Terrors of the Night*, London, William Jones, 1594, p. 4. George Herbert, 'The Church-porch', LXXVI, *The Temple*, Cambridge, 1633. Historians of affect, see William Bouwsma, *A Usable Past: Essays in European Cultural History*, Berkeley, University of California Press, 1990, pp. 19–73.

p. 163 Franz Kafka, *Letters to Milena*, London, Vintage, 1999, p. 22.

p. 164 Martha Wolfenstein and Nathan Leites, *Movies: A Psychological Study*, New York, Free Press, 1950, p. 200.

p. 169 Regrets of the day, see Samuel Tissot, *An Essay on the Disorders of People of Fashion*, London, 1771, p. 38.

p. 170 Nathaniel Kleitman, 'Studies in the physiology of sleep', *American Journal of Physiology*, 66, 1923, p. 67, quoted in Kroker, *The Sleep of Others*, op. cit., p. 216.

p. 175 Hartmann, *The Sleeping Pill*, op. cit., p. 136.

p. 176 Structural guilt, see M. West, 'Ancestral curses', in Jasper Griffin, ed., *Sophocles Revisited: Essays Presented to Sir Hugh Lloyd-Jones*, Oxford University Press, 1999, pp. 31–45. Sigmund Freud, *Totem and Taboo*, (1913), in *Totem and Taboo and Other Works*, Standard Edition, Vol. 13, London, Hogarth, 1955, pp. 1–161; Sigmund Freud, *Civilisation and Its Discontents* (1930), in *The Future of an Illusion, Civilisation and its Discontents, and Other Works*, Standard Edition, Vol. 21, London, Hogarth, 1961, pp. 64–145; Herman Nunberg, 'The sense of guilt and the need for punishment', *International Journal of Psychoanalysis*, 7, 1926, pp. 420–33.

p. 178 Jacques Lacan, *The Seminar of Jacques Lacan, Book VIII, Transference* (1960–61), ed. J.-A. Miller, Cambridge, Polity, 2015, p. 302.

p. 180 Margaret Mead and Frances Macgregor, *Growth and Culture*, New York, Putnam's, 1951, p. 96; see also Carol Worthman and Melissa Melby, 'Toward a comparative developmental ecology of human sleep', in Mary Carskadon, ed., *Adolescent Sleep Patterns*, Cambridge University Press, 2004, pp. 69–117.

p. 182 Martin Buber, 'Guilt and guilt feelings', *Psychiatry*, 20, 1957, pp. 114–29.

Acknowledgements

As I started researching this book, my sleep got much better, but by the end it was far worse. In contrast to other topics I have written about, sleep is just so little understood, and I have spent many, many hours awake trying to resolve some of its contradictions and problems. I don't think I've solved much in this book, but hope to have opened up some questions and troubled some received opinions, showing how we really need to think more about sleep and what happens within it. So much about sleep and dreaming remains unknown, and it is a genuinely exciting field of research, which can no doubt illuminate the underlying question of how our minds and bodies work, and the modes of their intersection.

Special thanks to Pat Blackett, Astrid Gessert, Olga Grotova and Mike Witcombe for their invaluable help with research, and to everyone else who has contributed to this book: Josh Appignanesi, Chloe Aridjis, Devorah Baum, Susie Boyt, Lina Brocchieri, David Corfield, Vincent Dachy, Marie Darrieussecq, Bryony Davies, Jean Duprat, Elanor Dymott, Camille Germanos, Anouchka Grose, Rachel Kneebone, Hanif Kureishi, Elliot Leader, Catherine Millot, Geneviève Morel, Susie Orbach, Boika Sokolova, Eleanor Tattersfield, Kristina Valendinova, Anabelle Vanier-Clement, and Jay Watts. Thank you to Julia Carne, Berjanet Jazani, Alexandra Langley, Anne

Worthington and everyone at the Centre for Freudian Analysis and Research, where we held a lively and inspiring conference on insomnia in 2017. At Hamish Hamilton, Simon Prosser was as ever an acute and sympathetic editor, and Hermione Thomson's comments were both helpful and enlightening. Tracy Bohan at Wylie is the most collected and savvy agent one could hope for, making the whole publishing process run smoothly and seamlessly. And thank you Mary, Jack, Iris and Clem for sharing your thoughts about this book – or at least, the fact that I was writing it – and tolerating the accumulation of sleep-related books, journals, offprints and manuals that now overrun almost every room in our house.

DARIAN LEADER

WHAT IS MADNESS?

What separates the sane from the mad? How hard or easy is it to tell them apart? And what if the difference is really between being mad and going mad?

In this landmark work Darian Leader undermines common conceptions of madness. Through case studies like that of the apparently 'normal' Harold Shipman, he shows that madness rarely conforms to the images we might expect. By exploring the idea of 'quiet madness' – that psychosis and an uneventful normal life are absolutely compatible – he argues that we must radically revise our understanding of madness.

'Provides valuable insights into how psychiatry can help those who have suffered psychosis to rebuild their lives' *Sunday Times*

'Witty, probing. A myth-busting diagnosis of the method in our madness' *Independent*

'Leader's insights could have radical consequences for the way we regard madness' *Daily Telegraph*

DARIAN LEADER

THE NEW BLACK

How hard or easy is it to tell what happens when we lose someone we love? A death, a separation or the break-up of a relationship are some of the hardest times we have to live through. We may fall into a nightmare of depression, lose the will to live and see no hope for the future. What matters at this crucial point is whether or not we are able to mourn.

In this important and groundbreaking book, acclaimed psychoanalyst and writer Darian Leader urges us to look beyond the catch-all concept of depression to explore the deeper, unconscious ways in which we respond to the experience of loss. In so doing, we can loosen the grip it may have upon our lives.

'His orthodox, psychoanalytical approach produces an unpredictable, occasionally brilliant book. *The New Black* is a mixture of Freudian text, clinical assessments and Leader's own brand of gentle wisdom' *Herald*

'Compelling and important . . . an engrossing and wise book' **Hanif Kureishi**

'There are many self-help books on the market . . . *The New Black* is a book that might actually help' *Independent*

He just wanted a decent book to read ...

Not too much to ask, is it? It was in 1935 when Allen Lane, Managing Director of Bodley Head Publishers, stood on a platform at Exeter railway station looking for something good to read on his journey back to London. His choice was limited to popular magazines and poor-quality paperbacks – the same choice faced every day by the vast majority of readers, few of whom could afford hardbacks. Lane's disappointment and subsequent anger at the range of books generally available led him to found a company – and change the world.

'We believed in the existence in this country of a vast reading public for intelligent books at a low price, and staked everything on it'
Sir Allen Lane, 1902–1970, founder of Penguin Books

The quality paperback had arrived – and not just in bookshops. Lane was adamant that his Penguins should appear in chain stores and tobacconists, and should cost no more than a packet of cigarettes.

Reading habits (and cigarette prices) have changed since 1935, but Penguin still believes in publishing the best books for everybody to enjoy. We still believe that good design costs no more than bad design, and we still believe that quality books published passionately and responsibly make the world a better place.

So wherever you see the little bird – whether it's on a piece of prize-winning literary fiction or a celebrity autobiography, political tour de force or historical masterpiece, a serial-killer thriller, reference book, world classic or a piece of pure escapism – you can bet that it represents the very best that the genre has to offer.

Whatever you like to read – trust Penguin.

read more
www.penguin.co.uk